JENNE DAVIS

I'm the head honcho over at Clitical.Com, but I see myself as more of a gate keeper than the webmistress. Whilst I do own several whips I'm generally not the one wielding them; I would rather spend my time writing about them and so many other things. I believe that sex is about sharing and open communication. When I'm not writing I can be found researching new techniques, reading, and on occasions cooking for my long suffering Hubby and kids.

www.clitical.com

@CliticalJenne

The Clitical Guide to Female Self-Pleasure

How to Please Yourself So Your Partner Can Too

JENNE DAVIS

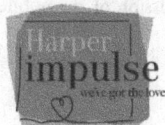

Harper*Impulse* an imprint of
HarperCollins*Publishers* Ltd
1 London Bridge Street
London SE1 9GF

www.harpercollins.co.uk

A Paperback Original 2015

First published in Great Britain in ebook format by Harper*Impulse* 2015

Cover images © Shutterstock.com

Jenne Davis asserts the moral right
to be identified as the author of this work

A catalogue record for this book is
available from the British Library

ISBN: 978-0-00-814642-9

This novel is entirely a work of fiction.
The names, characters and incidents portrayed in it are
the work of the author's imagination. Any resemblance to
actual persons, living or dead, events or localities is
entirely coincidental.

Automatically produced by Atomik ePublisher from Easypress

To my amazing daughter and friends, who never allowed me to give up on my dreams, or myself. Never stop dreaming or using your imagination because you never know where those crazy dreams might take you...

Introduction

Female masturbation, self-love, self-pleasure – call it what you will. For most women masturbation is often their first exploration into the wonderful, but sometimes seemingly daunting world of sexuality. Personally, I can't think of a better place to start than by having sex with yourself – can you?

Like many women, my first hurdle, when it came to masturbation, was learning it was okay to touch myself. I recall reasoning that it was my own body and belonged to no one except myself. That said, I went through the pangs of wondering if I would be condemned for practising, well, you know, 'that' kind of touching. That word, which was rarely, if ever, uttered in my, and, I suspect, most homes across the world. Yes, that word! Masturbation!

I grew up in a time when masturbation was rarely mentioned in the media and was definitely something that you never told anyone you had tried. Even your closest friend, for the most part, was off limits, because they might just tell someone else. I recall the stress of keeping that secret so well – and I'm about to approach fifty this year. The truth was, like many teens, once I discovered that touching my private parts made me feel deliciously good, it was as though I never wanted to stop. I devised secret ways to touch myself. I spent countless hours in my bedroom, just discovering the pleasure that my own body was capable of producing and yet that pleasure would often be tinged with guilt. Guilt that somehow what I was doing was, in fact, inherently wrong, but no one ever really took the time to tell me why it was so wrong. After all, it wasn't as if anyone ever took me aside and said, 'If you touch yourself you are going to hell', but still, I felt that guilt.

In some ways I wish that guilt had never existed and, to be honest, I hope that this book will help you put that guilt aside so you can simply enjoy what is, after all, a safe and wonderful teaching aid when it comes to sexuality: masturbation.

Society, for the most part, has come to realize, that self-love is probably the safest form of sexual expression there is. It's also a wonderful learning tool and by learning what turns us on, and in some cases turn us off, we are not only better individuals but we, as females, make in many cases much better partners and lovers.

I don't consider myself an expert when it comes to the art of self-pleasure, and I don't aspire to be. I can tell you I am a life-long masturbator and glad to be able to call myself that, hoping to be able to practice until I am well into my old, old age.

Over the years, I have come to think of masturbation as an ever-evolving form of sexuality, and there is no one technique that is guaranteed to bring you the pot of gold at the end of the rainbow, the infamous orgasm. I'm not sure how I managed to achieve my first orgasm at the age of 15. I was just playing around with my new-found toy (my body) and it happened, but once it had happened, I wanted it to happen again and again. Maybe if I had known what I had experienced back then it might have helped. It might also have helped had I thought about taking note of what I was touching, when and where, but that has always been the most

2

wonderful part of the entire masturbation experience for me: not quite knowing why, when, or where the next orgasm was going to come. The mechanism that caused me to orgasm was just part of the bigger picture and I developed something of a lust for the answer to the question why. Why does this feel so good? Then came the how, as in how can I make this feel even better, followed by the when and where would be the best time to do this, in order to make it better? Could it even get any better?

So I set off on a quest, which at that time seemed to be of epic proportions, to find the answer to those questions. That was when I discovered that this was to be no easy task. No one talked about masturbation back then – it was a dark secret, a sin to be hidden away at all costs, because even though you could talk about what you did with your partner/boyfriend last Saturday night, talking about what you did to yourself, amongst even your closest girl-friends, was akin to admitting you were less of a person because you didn't have, or couldn't get, a boyfriend. In other words, you were the biggest loser on the block. Sex with yourself must be second-rate sex, after all, which to me, never did make any sense. But it was, and still is in many cases to this day, the accepted norm when we talk about solo sex.

Back then there was no Internet, no real sex-toy boutiques, or at least not the type that most women would ever be seen outside, let alone leaving, lest you were spied by the local neighborhood noses, or, worse still, your so-called friends. Like many women of the time, I got my sexual information from the copies of the *Penthouse* that my dad had stashed beneath the clothes in his closet. Sex education at schools was basic, to say the least, and the only thing I really learned from those lessons was that sex was embarrassing and something to be made fun of. I never felt that way about solo or partnered sex, though. How could something that made me feel this good be so bad, after all?

With the advent of the Internet and the fact that I could communicate with the entire universe and beyond, it became easier to
learn about sex, yet somehow it always felt as though solo sex
was partnered sex's ugly sister. You know – that one member of
the family who is always at weddings and funerals but sits in the
corner because no one from the family really wants them there. I
began to question how this could be so. How on earth could that
be wrong when you are simply loving yourself? At the same time,
women were being taught that we could do, or have, anything we
wanted. We had the right to demand orgasms from our partners,
it was our birthright and if they couldn't give us one as prescribed
by the pages of *Cosmopolitan*, then he didn't deserve us.

As my quest for answers continued, I became almost more
confused. Why was partnered sex the hallowed ground? Was there
no place in sexuality for solo sex other than as the ugly sister?
I'd always had that strange tinge of guilt that came after an often
mammoth session of self-loving, but, darn, if it felt this good how
on earth could it be bad?

Anyway, I discovered the Internet, but more than that, I discovered
erotic writing. I found a way to channel my own guilt at enjoying
sex, and especially solo sex, so much, into my characters. As I wrote
more and posted them onto the Net I began to form the idea of a
website: a site where women could feel safe asking questions about
sex, love, and everything in between, and so could their partners.
In the year 2000, thanks to a partnership with Art, the wonderful
webmaster over at EroticStories.com, that dream became a reality.
As so often happens in life, my love of solo sex and my search
for answers to my quest became something that was ever more
prominent on our new website: Clitical.com

Over the years Clitical has become a labor of love, some might
say a labor of self- love. As time went by, I realized that self-love

4

encompasses so much more than a simple technique. It's way more than just a means to an end. Self-pleasure is about learning to love your sexual self. It's a safe form of sexual expression, with a few exceptions, and it can take your partnered sex to a whole new level if you open your mind.

As Clitical has grown it has seen many redesigns, but the core of the site remains the same: a place where women can learn about sex, especially self-love, not just from me, but from their peers. Over the years we have amassed a huge collection of female visitors' masturbation techniques, fantasies, and a whole lot more besides. I've been asked all manner of questions, sexual and otherwise. I've met some of the coolest people on the planet, and all thanks to a quest to answer the question of why self- pleasure is the ugly sister of partnered sex. I've discovered the many facets that make up human sexuality, that no two individuals are alike, and that there is no right or wrong way to pleasure yourself or a partner, only the way that works for you. That journey of discovery is ultimately what this book is about. As you take that journey yourself, I hope that you will find this book will help you discover what works for you and sometimes what doesn't, helps you feel less afraid to try something new, to just jump in and discover, because of all the things I've learned, the most important one is: you have to live in your moment, this moment, the one that is happening right now.

CHAPTER 1

Female Anatomy

Love Thyself

Getting to know your own anatomy is the basic foundation for all sexual encounters, whether solo or partnered. Until you are comfortable within your own skin, touching your own skin and seeing it as not just part of your body but as a part of your sexual self, it's unlikely that you will be comfortable sexually.

Most of us think of the sexual parts of our body as being our breasts, vulvas, and vaginas. Occasionally we throw in our butts, for good measure, but our entire body has the potential to offer us sexual pleasure if we know how to tap into the secrets that it holds. This chapter is designed to help you see that sexually you are much more than those three, or possibly four, body parts, depending on how you look at it.

Let's Get One Thing Straight!

Before we go any further, though, let's get one thing straight from the get-go...

Vulvas are not vaginas. Despite the fact that they both begin with the letter V and are part of one another and, more importantly, part of you, they perform very different functions when it comes to sex. Vaginas are the inner part of the vulva, which is the outside part of your female sexual anatomy. Yet so many of us don't know that simple difference – and I'm not just referring to the male species here – women are equally guilty when they talk about their vulvas and refer to them as their vaginas.

If you enjoy clitoral pleasure, and, yes, we will get to discussing your clitoris in the next chapter, then you are touching your vulva. If you enjoy penetrative sex, then you are using your vagina. There is a difference and it is important to understand the difference; learning to use the correct term is a great way to show others that you understand your own body as well.

Are You Sitting Comfortably?

The other reason why many of us feel uncomfortable when it comes to masturbation is that we are often taught that our vulvas are something that should always be hidden, which is admittedly not helped by the fact that they are securely nestled between our upper thighs, and are, in fact, well, hidden. Cotton knickers or panties are placed there and we are told only to make sure that we wear clean panties each day. I clearly recall my own mother declaring that this was in case I was ever in a car accident. Looking back, that was a silly statement, but at the time I took her warning seriously as I'm sure many other little girls did and still do.

I tried to recall an instance where I was actually told not to ever show my hidden or private parts to a boy, and I really can't. It was just something that you never did – if you were a good girl. When you sat down and were wearing a skirt, the norm was to ensure that no part of your privates was exposed to the stare of a guy. Again, no specific instructions may have ever been given; it was something you simply learned unconsciously. After all, they were your 'private' parts. Now, I'm not suggesting that you go around wearing no panties or show your vulva to the next guy that walks into your office or workplace. I'm just trying to illustrate where we may have learned the idea that our vulvas are for our lovers' eyes only and until then shall remain private at all costs.

A Fish by Any Other Name

Another reason that you may feel discomfort when talking about, or looking at, your own genitals is that rarely are our genitals referred to by their correct names. Instead they are referred to as 'private parts', or worst still, 'fish', 'star fish', 'love taco', 'meat curtains', 'twat', or some other equally demeaning name. None of which helps us to get comfortable with them in any way, shape, or form. Many of these names came from an era when talking about sex was frowned upon. It could be said that this is still true, but things are getting better and by learning the correct terms to use when it comes to your own anatomy, you are part of the solution, not part of the problem, so to speak.

More than the Sum of Four

Many women only think of sex in terms of our breasts, buttocks, and, of course, our vulvas as being the sexual part of our beings and that is something of a shame. As we will see in the next chapter, the biggest sexual organ we have is, in fact, our brain, but when we turn our mental thoughts into physical actions amazing things can happen and our entire bodies can become our very own playgrounds of pleasure.

So, let's start by taking a look at our anatomy from top to bottom – so to speak! For the exercises I've included in this chapter you might find that a hand-held mirror will come in handy, so now would be the perfect time to find one.

Skin

Your skin is, in fact, the largest organ in your body and it contains at least five types of receptors that respond to both pain and touch. An average adult's skin spans 21 square feet, weighs nine pounds, and contains more than 11 miles of blood vessels. Your skin releases as much as three gallons of sweat a day in hot weather. There are a couple of areas that don't sweat and these are the beds of your nails, the margins of your lips, the tip of the penis (if you have one), and your eardrums. Who knew, right?

We tend to take the fact that we have skin as it's, well, just always been there. If you take a minute to look at your skin in a slightly different light you will realize what an important part it can play when it comes to both solo and partnered sex.

Exercise:
In blind people, the brain's visual cortex is rewired to respond to stimuli received via touch and hearing. This allows the blind person to actually 'see' the world through touch and sound. If you don't believe me, try this simple experiment and 'see' the world and your skin in a different light.

Begin by either turning the lights off or simply placing a blind-fold over your eyes, making sure you really can't peek out. Now take some time exploring your own skin. Notice the touches you make. What do you see? By applying more or less pressure you can experiment with the results of one study that revealed that the Meissner corpuscles – touch receptors that are concentrated in the fingertips and palms, lips and tongue, nipples, penis and clitoris – respond to a pressure of just 20 milligrams, or the weight of a fly. Science is amazing, isn't it?

Hair
As silly as it might sound, your hair is an important part of your identity and though we rarely think of it as being sexy, nothing could be further from the truth. We tend to think of hair and sex

in terms of partnered sex, but it doesn't have to be that way. Try this simple exercise to see what I mean:

Exercise:
Take a small clump of hair and run your fingers through it, over it, and even give it a gentle tug. Now do this with your eyes closed and see if the feelings it produces change. I'm willing to bet that it will. The chances are it became much more sexual when you closed your eyes than when they were open.

Ears
We rarely think of our ears in terms of sexuality, but the truth is your ears can be a huge part of your solo sex repertoire if only you would let them. Some women can get turned on simply by touching their own ears, but this is not true in all cases. However, it's worth trying, as they say – nothing ventured nothing gained – and the outcome might surprise you. Of course, the thing we generally use our ears for is to hear what is around us. The things that surround us can often be surprisingly sexual, if only we listen to them.

Exercise:
If you watch porn, start by finding your favorite scene. Now watch it without the sound. Now watch it again with the sound on and your eyes closed. Notice the differences between the experiences. You could also try investing in an audio erotic book and listen to it with your eyes shut (unless, of course, you happen to be driving at the time of listening.)

Lips
Our lips are packed with nerve ending that send many signals to our brains – some sexual and others not. It's not easy to kiss yourself, but it's not impossible, if you think about it. You can kiss your own hand – you can even kiss your own breasts if the

10

mood so takes you. After all, it's your body and you are free to explore it any way you like.

Exercise:
Try simply running your tongue over your lips: slowly, now very slowly. Notice the way your body reacts as you do this. Does it turn you on or have no effect? Everyone has different reactions to everything and especially to the way you touch it.

Tongue

We are what we eat, as they say, and eating something can be a very sexy experience. Our tongues are packed with taste buds that allow us to feel and interrupt the sensations caused by sweetness, bitterness, saltiness, sourness, and umami. Different tastes can, in fact, cause our bodies to react in sexual ways. I'm sure you are familiar with the saying 'sex is better than chocolate', but are all too aware that there are times when the opposite is true. By discovering which tastes you enjoy when you are solo it is possible to turn what you eat into a sexual experience.

Exercise:
Try eating some ice cream. Pick a flavor that you know you enjoy, or if you are feeling a little more adventurous, pick one that you have never tried. Now settle down and use a spoon – feed yourself that ice cream, slowly... very slowly. Concentrate on the sensations that the taste produces within you. You are likely to react to the coolness of the ice cream at first, but now try licking the ice cream from the back of the spoon. Again, move slowly and deliberately. It may help if you close your eyes as you concentrate solely on the sensations. I've had some great solo ice-cream escapades over the years. It's all about changing your perception of what you are doing. You're not just eating, you're tasting, enjoying, and – most of all – feeling.

Neck

There are times when I swear my neck is in some way directly connected to my vulva and clitoris. Whether I'm simply touching it gently with my hand or my partner is with their lips or hand, I can't help but get a little moister between my thighs and my thoughts turn to sex. I'm sure I'm not the only one who has this connection, and you can find out whether your neck reacts the same way as mine does by trying this simple but effective exercise.

Exercise:

Try running your fingertips across the nape of your neck. Vary the pressure you use as you explore this often-neglected part of your body. You can try experimenting by using various objects such as silk scarves, feathers, and anything else you have at hand – to see the effects the sensations have on you. They might just surprise you!

Shoulders and Arms

Both of these items are rarely thought of as sexy, but they should never be discounted as such when it comes to solo sex.

Exercise:

Try touching your shoulder and arms with either your opposite hand or a variety of objects. These objects can run the gamut from silk scarves to pieces of wood. Try varying the force or pressure that you apply to these areas and spend some time noticing how your body reacts to them.

Hands

If there is one area of your body that you might want to start thinking of in terms of a sexual tool, it would likely be your hands. Yes, you read that right! Take a second to think this through if this fact is throwing you off. Your hands touch, your hands feel, your hands are amazing. Even if you choose to use a sexual toy or tool, you will likely have to hold it with, well, your hand – or hands. Hopefully you are starting to see what I mean, here. The great thing about your hands is that they cost nothing, are always – ermmm – handy, and have the ability to bring you lots of sexual pleasure, if you would only let them.

Exercise:
We tend to think of sexual touch in terms of fingertips, when we can, and probably should, be using the entire surface of our hands. You can apply this logic to any of the exercises and techniques that are included in this book. If a technique calls for you to use your fingertips, there are no rules to say you can't try the same thing with the palm of your hands, be it a movement or applying pressure.

Breasts
For most women, and, let's face it, men, breasts are something that hold a special place in their hearts when it comes to sex. Breasts are made up of mostly fatty and connective tissue. Just like most other body parts, breasts come in many different sizes, shapes, and colors. They can be the same size and shape, but oftentimes one breast may look a little different than the other. The breasts and nipples may enlarge in the days prior to a woman's period and may grow extra sensitive during this time – as well as during (and after) pregnancy.

In other words, breasts are somewhat complicated and then you can add in the fact that according to one study around 50 per cent of women enjoy breast stimulation, whilst the others simply tolerate it to please a partner. The good news here is we are talking about solo sex and there is no one else to please but you! According to studies conducted by Masters and Johnson and the Kinsey Institute, a small percentage of women can actually have an orgasm from breast stimulation alone. Interestingly enough, in a Kinsey Institute experiment on 8,000 women, only 11 per cent said they stimulated their own breasts during masturbation. I say that it's time we changed that percentage and I wish more women would explore their breasts as well as the rest of their bodies during a masturbation session.

Exercise:

Start out by touching your breasts using long, circular strokes, starting at the bottom of your breasts. Slowly graze your skin with your fingers as you circle the outer perimeter of your breasts. With each revolution of your breast, move just a little closer to the center of your breast, spiraling inward ever so slightly. For every two movements closer to your breasts, take one small movement outward. Continue with slow, spiraling strokes toward your nipples. As you near the nipple with one hand, stop and begin the same process with your other one. Take your time touching your breasts – make this whole process take at least 10 to15 minutes. When you do finally get to your nipple, you may well find yourself in ecstasy.

Nipples

Did you know that it's possible for a woman to achieve orgasm solely through nipple play? It's true! This doesn't happen for every woman, but certain women can have genital orgasms that are caused by intense nipple stimulation. About one in 18 people are born with a third nipple and during the Middle Ages if you did have a third nipple you would have been branded a witch, which would likely have meant you would have been burned at the stake. Fortunately we live in the 21st century and those days are done. That said, many people still have many misconceptions about their nipples, so let's try to put them to rest, shall we?

In case you aren't aware, the circular pigmented area around your nipple is called the 'aureola'. They range in color from pale yellow to almost black, and are always darker than the skin that makes up the breast. This is so it's easier for a baby to locate them. Generally the older you are the bigger your aureolas will be. Hairs do not grow on your actual nipple, preferring to grow on your aureola, and are not bad. Whilst an erect nipple can be a sign that you are feeling sexually aroused there are other reasons they may become erect, including the fact that it's darn cold.

Exercise:
Lube the tips of the thumb and index finger of your dominant hand. If you don't have any lube handy, you can simply lick your fingers to moisten them before beginning. Now place your fingers directly across from each other on opposite ends of the outer aureola. Start at the outer part of the aureola and move your finger and thumb toward each other. As they reach the nipple, roll the nipple in a twirling motion between your fingertip and the tip of your thumb. Now, repeat the technique, starting at a different spot on the outside of the aureola. This will tease the nipple by creating anticipation and desire. Where you take things from here is, well, in your own hands.

Stomach or Belly
In men, this area is often referred to as the 'treasure trail', and this is the way I like to think of it when it comes to solo sex. Some women will find that when they are sexually aroused their stomach, or belly, area becomes too sensitive to touch, whilst others enjoy exploring this area and view it as foreplay before they reach the promised land of their mons, or the top of their vulva.

Exercise:
Spend some time playing with your belly once you are sexually aroused. Does it feel good as you allow your hand to travel downward toward your mons or does it have the opposite effect? Try varying the pressure, direction, and width of your touch and see if that makes a difference.

The Mons Veneris

Your Mons Veneris is located below your abdomen or belly, but above your vulva. It's the area of fatty tissue that covers your pubic bone and is designed to cushion/protect your pubic bone from the impact of intercourse. You might find it to be very sensitive when you are aroused, but this is not always the case. In its natural state it is covered by pubic hair, which is believed to trap the natural aroma of your vagina. Of course, if you've shaved it, this area will be clear of pubic hair.

Exercise:

Once you are sexually aroused, or 'horny', why not try using different touches over and around the area of your mons area. Some women enjoy a tapping technique and the only way to discover if this works for you is to, well, try it. Vary the rhythm and also the pressure you apply, and also you can experiment with not just your fingertips but also the entire palm of your hand to discover what you like or dislike.

Inner Thighs

Let's face it, most good touches eventually lead to the inner thighs, as this is where you will find your vulva nestled, but before you get there, why not spend some time circling around the sensitive skin that you will find nestled between your thighs. As we rarely touch our inner thighs, you will likely find they respond to your touch in a positive way and are worth spending some time getting to know.

Exercise:

As with your stomach or belly, spend some time getting to know your inner thighs. You may enjoy using a lighter touch here, as this is an area of your body that rarely gets any attention via touch. You can also vary the type of touch, by using a silk scarf, wearing woolen gloves or anything you might have handy. Experiment until you find what works for you.

16

Vulva

The vulva is the term that refers to all of a woman's externally visible genitalia. Many people commonly make the mistake of referring to the vulva as the vagina, but the vagina is actually just the internal canal. Everything you can see from the outside is referred to as the vulva. One of the most interesting things about the vulva is that they are like fingerprints; they are each as individual as you are. I've yet to find any evidence that CSI has found a way to produce a reliable vulva print as yet, but it is an interesting idea nonetheless.

Exercise:

Grab a hand mirror, get naked, get comfortable, and examine your vulva up close and personal. Locate all of your important parts. You wouldn't believe how many women have never engaged in self-exploration. There are many reasons you should do so. First, it helps if you can locate, identify, and name all your body parts when you go to see your doctor. This may be a bit uncomfortable for you, but it is definitely less embarrassing than trying to explain to your doctor that your 'kitty' hurts, and it's definitely more effective than telling the doctor that you hurt 'down there'. It's also good to know what your vulva looks like in its healthy state, so you can identify problems if things don't look quite right.

Labia Majora

The labia majora are designed with one purpose – to enclose and protect your other external reproductive organs. Your labia majora are also often referred to as the 'outer lips' and are the fat, fleshy lips that extend the length of your vulva. Like most things associated with the vulva they will vary greatly in size from woman to woman and there is no 'right' or 'wrong' size, with some being more visible than others. Unless you shave them, they are covered in a coating of pubic hair from the time you reach puberty.

Your labia majora contain sweat and oil glands that are responsible for the familiar scent that is associated with sexual arousal. For many women this scent can cause anxiety but, to be honest, for many men this scent can be extremely attractive. A healthy vagina produces a slightly musky smell when you are aroused and this is a normal part of the arousal process and should not worry you.

Exercise:
Lie on your back with your legs spread wide open. I like to prop myself up with a pillow when I do this as I like to see what I'm doing, but that's a personal choice. Now take some lube and apply it to your thumb and forefinger, pinch your outer labia together, and stroke them up and down. As always, concentrate solely on the feelings this produces within your body.

Labia Minora
Your labia minora, or inner lips, are designed to act like a pair of swinging doors guarding the entrance to the vagina and the urethra, the tube that leads from the bladder. Your labia minora are much thinner than your labia majora and even more sensitive. They also contain erectile tissue made up of clusters of tiny blood vessels, which means they become slightly stiffer (though not as stiff as your clitoris) when you are aroused.

Like many other things about your body, inner lips come in an infinite number of varieties. Some are tiny and sit neatly between your outer lips, while others will be much larger and hang out from below the outer lips. Some are thick and some are thin, but whatever shape or size they may be, they are all hairless and sensitive to the touch. As you become aroused you will likely find they change color due to the fact that they fill with blood when you are more turned on.

18

Exercise:

Remember that hand-held mirror I asked you to collect at the beginning of this chapter? Now is the time to find it and put it to good use again. Take some time to get comfortable and position the mirror so you have a good view of your vulva. I find it easier to do this by propping the mirror against the wall or a pillow and then sitting in front of it. Now take a good look at your inner lips, notice everything about them, for example their size and color. Now take one of your inner lips between your finger and thumb and start massaging it gently. Alternate between your two lips and notice any changes as you massage them. You will likely find that the color changes as you become more aroused.

The Urethra

The urethra is the medical term for your urinary opening or your pee hole. As the more common name suggests, this is where you pee from. The urethral opening is located between your clitoris and your vagina opening and is hidden between the labia minora. Its exact location will vary from woman to woman and it may or may not be clearly visible. The opening itself is a vertical, slit-like, or egg-shaped opening, that is around 4–5mm in diameter.

Your urethra's main function in life is to give you somewhere to pee from. In some women it is possible to trigger an orgasm by stimulating the opening to the urethra but as a general rule it's not a great idea to place anything inside your urethra as this can cause a plethora of problems.

Exercise:

The urethra, as I said before, is where you pee from, and although it's not really thought of as a sexual thing it can be used as part of an exercise to strengthen your PC muscles, which will help with your sex life as a whole. The first thing to do is identify the PC muscle. The next time you go to the bathroom, sit on the toilet with your legs spread apart and see if you can stop and start the flow of urine without moving your legs or squeezing your buttocks together. If you're doing it right you'll feel an internal flexing and tightening beneath your bladder, in which case, congratulate yourself! You just found your PC muscle! A word of caution here. This is a great way of finding your PC muscle, but once you've identified the muscle, then make sure you aren't peeing when you actually begin practicing the kegels as this can cause bladder infections. So now you've found your PC muscle, just follow these simple steps and you are doing your kegels!

1. Breathe normally.
2. Contract your PC muscle.
3. Hold for a count of five.
4. Relax your PC muscle.
5. Repeat ten times.

Clitoris

The clitoris is the only organ in the human body that has no known purpose other than producing sexual pleasure. You can find the clitoris at the 12:00 position of your vulva. It's located near the top of the vulva and may be hidden under the labia and/ or clitoral hood. The head of the clitoris, or clitoral glans, is the small pea-sized bud of smooth, spongy, erectile tissue located at the top of the labia minora. It is covered, either partially or completely, by the clitoral hood – a flap of skin that looks like a hood over a little head. The clitoral hood is designed to protect the head of the clitoris, which may become erect and protrude from the clitoral hood when you are fully turned on.

However, the visible head of the clitoris is just the tip of the iceberg. When someone uses the phrase 'the tip of the iceberg', it refers to the fact that as much as seven-eighths of the iceberg's mass is under water, leaving only a small portion exposed. The clitoris is very much like an iceberg in that only the small glans is visible to us, but it actually extends into the body. The entire clitoris resembles a four-inch wishbone. It extends from the external and visible pea-sized tip, up the shaft, and into the body.

Just as penises come in all shapes and sizes so do clitorises and while the average size of the clitoris is about one-quarter of an inch in diameter, it is possible to have a clitoris that can measure up to two and a half inches in length and one inch in diameter. When they are this large they bear a striking resemblance to a small penis, which is not really so surprising when you learn that the penis and clitoris are made up of the same tissues and develop from the same tissue when they are in the fetus. As with breasts, the clitoris will vary in size from woman to woman, and a small clitoris does not impact a woman's ability to orgasm.

Exercise:
Take a hand-held mirror and take another look at your vulva. Really concentrate on finding your clitoris this time. Not just your clitoral head, but your entire clitoris, which includes the shaft that runs along your inner labia. Now spend a little time touching just one side of your clitoral shaft at first, then the other. The fascinating thing about the clitoral shaft is that many women will report more sensitivity on one side than the other. As you stroke each side of the shaft, take note of how your clitoris reacts to each touch. If you have a large clitoral hood, then the chances are you will see the clitoris or pea-shaped object begin to peek out as you become more aroused. If you have a small clitoral hood, this might be a little less pronounced, but look a little closer and get familiar with your clitoris.

Vagina
The vagina performs many functions. Not only does it accept the penis during sex, captures sperm during ejaculation, and acts as a

pathway for an egg, it also provides sexual pleasure, allows us to give birth and also to have periods. The vagina is the term that refers to the internal workings of the vulva and, as I have said before, people often confuse the two. Vulva outside: vagina inside.

Like your eye, your vagina is a self-cleaning organ. No, it doesn't cry, but it does produce fluids that will cause it to naturally cleanse itself. It is a muscular barrel that measures in at around three or four inches long when you are not turned on. This might not sound very long, given that the average penis measures in at around five inches, but this is where the magic of the vagina really begins. Once you are turned on, or 'aroused', to give it its correct term, your vagina has the ability to expand. Think of it as a piece of elastic, if you will. This elastic nature is what allows a woman to accommodate pretty much any size of penis. It also allows us to give birth, although this process is slightly different from the one above. Your vagina is angled upward at around a 65-degree angle, which is, indecently, the angle that the average penis sits at once it is erect. Unlike some popular myths would have us believe, the vagina is not a wide-open, gaping hole. It's actually a collapsed space that contracts and expands when excited or penetrated. When you are turned on your vagina stretches out as you become more excited. In addition, your cervix and uterus will pull up and backward to allow more space for penetration, whilst the back of the vagina balloons out to create even more space. When you are not aroused your vagina resembles a collapsed hose.

If you took a look inside your vagina, you would find it is pink, glistening, and has folds, called 'rugea', which give your vagina a ribbed texture. When you are younger these folds are more pronounced, but as you grow older they gradually disappear. When you become turned on, your vagina begins to lubricate itself and forms what look like beads of sweat all over its walls. The first third of your vagina is where you will find two-thirds of the nerve endings that reside there. So, as a general rule, the first two inches of your vagina are the tightest and the most sensitive when you are being penetrated. This is due to the fact that this area will fill with blood and become engorged.

Despite popular belief, you cannot accurately determine how turned on a woman is just by her vaginal wetness. It's possible to be highly aroused and have a completely dry vagina. Most of the time your ability to self-lubricate will be affected by a couple of things: your level of estrogen or other hormones can greatly change at certain times, such as, for example, if you are stressed, sick, have a poor diet, or depending on where you are with your menstrual cycle. As is well documented that as you reach the menopause vaginal dryness is much more common due to your body producing less estrogen, but this is easily overcome by adding some personal lubricant into the mix.

Exercise:
If you are comfortable with inserting a finger into your vagina then you can try this exercise. If you aren't, it's fine to wait until you are comfortable with doing so.

Place your finger into your vagina and feel around. I swear it won't bite. Take a moment to get used to both the feeling of your vagina being filled and also how your vagina feels.

Butt
So, I know what you're thinking! Why on earth would I put this into a book about female masturbation? The simple answer is: everyone has a butt and although, it's true, that it is always lagging behind, it can be a source of great foreplay when it comes to solo sex.

Exercise:
Have you ever tried slapping your butt, either gently or with greater

force? Just try it and you might just be surprised by the way your body responds to a slap when you are in the right frame of mine to be sexy and flirty with yourself. Try varying the pressure you use and see which type of pressure, if any, has an effect on you.

Anus and Perineum

Since time began, the anus has been accepted as an erogenous zone. The walls of your anus are packed jam-full of nerve endings and can provide a great deal of pleasure. The other part of your anatomy that you may gain pleasure from playing with is your perineum, which is located between your vaginal opening and your anus. This area also contains many, many nerve and can be very pleasurable to touch. Of course the anus is an area that is generally associated with poo, and for good reason, as this is where your body expels its waste. There are a couple of precautions you can, and should, take if you consider playing with your anus, especially anal penetration. I would strongly recommend that you invest in some latex gloves and make sure your fingernails are trimmed before you begin any type of anal play. The other is that the anus, unlike the vagina, does not self-lubricate and a good water-based lube can make any form of penetration a more pleasurable experience, and a safer one, as it is possible to tear the delicate muscles of the sphincter.

Exercise:

If you want to see if anal masturbation might be for you, I suggest you grab those latex gloves I just told you to buy, unless of course you have a latex allergy, and some of that water-based lube, and begin to explore. Start by pressing against your perineum and see how your body reacts. The most important thing to remember with any type of anal play is that you need to relax, especially if you decide to try penetration. If you do want to go further, start by exploring your anal opening, and then gently push your finger up and inside yourself. Start gently and with plenty of lube. If it hurts, then I suggest you stop, as you are too tense to receive your finger or even the top of your finger.

Calves

For many guys your calves can be a huge turn-on. It's the one reason that there are so many pictures of women wearing high heels. High heels accentuate your calves, and if you don't believe me, grab a pair of heels, head for the nearest full-length mirror and take a look at your calves with and without the heels on your feet. Now, can you see the difference?

Exercise:

Try wearing heels that you are comfortable wearing when you are getting ready for a solo session. If you are not someone who normally wears heels you will likely feel different and as you walk past a mirror you might well find yourself admiring your legs, and seeing them in a different light.

Feet and Toes

I will state for the record here that my toes and feet do not have a sexual bone in them, but this is not true for many women. Just as some men focus on their partner's feet and toes, some women find touching theirs can be a pleasurable experience. Others, like myself, don't, but you will never know unless you try.

Exercise:

Start by wetting your hands, and especially your fingertips, and spend some time playing with your feet and toes. Imagine your partner's tongue lapping over and between your toes as you explore with your fingertips and see what reactions you garner from your own feet and toes.

Conclusion:

Knowing your own anatomy can be a great way to start not only understanding how your body works sexually, but also what you may or may not enjoy whilst you are playing with a partner. The exercises above are just suggestions to help you get comfortable with your own body, but if you are not comfortable trying any of them, please feel free to ignore them until you are ready. This is your body and the great thing about owning it is that you can, and should, take things at your own pace. The idea, as I've said before, is for you to be able to become comfortable within your own skin. Once you have achieved that goal, the sky, as they say, is the limit!

CHAPTER 2

Masturbation: A Brief History

Where Did It All Begin?

It's quite likely that men and women have been masturbating since the beginning of time. In order to understand just why and how masturbation became partnered sex's ugly sister, we need to travel back in time. So I climbed into my own version of the Tardis a few years ago and travelled back into history. What follows are my findings as to why we have both the myths and stigma that may have, to some degree, dissipated, but that still hold many women back from enjoying all the pleasures their bodies are capable of achieving.

Beginning of Time: The Bible Edition

Before you get mad at me, I swear I'm not trying to be provocative here with that particular title, but it's hard to deny that religion and the belief that masturbation is wrong go hand in hand and the only way to discover why is to go back in time and find out. It would be remiss of me not to take a look at how these two things are linked.

It is often commonly assumed that *The Bible* specifically forbids masturbation. This belief has grown, in no small part, thanks to the story of Onan. Onan's story can be found in the book of Genesis, and to be more specific, chapter thirty-eight. In this chapter, Onan was required to marry his brother's widow and, more importantly, to provide her with a child who would then inherit his brother's estate. This was the Jewish practice at the time *The Bible* was penned.

Now if we look at the annotated *Bible* passage it, in fact, reads that since Onan knew that the offspring would not be his, he spilled his semen on the ground whenever he went to his brother's wife, so that he could give no offspring to his brother.

Onan was not put to death because he was masturbating but because he was practicing the withdrawal method of birth control. He did this in order to avoid fathering a child who would never legally be his.

It would not be until the 18th century that Onan's story would be interpreted by theologians of the time, as it is often now understood to mean that masturbation was not something that should ever be practiced. We will get to the 18th century in a little while, though. We have a few other centuries and continents that we need to travel to and through before we can truly understand the history of masturbation and the myths that have resulted.

Ancient China
Philosophers and doctors in Ancient China both held the belief that ejaculation from masturbation was a waste of what was, and still is, referred to as 'chi'. Chi was believed to be a form of energy that was vital to life, and that wasting it was never in the best interests of the patient or the person as a whole. In some of the first-ever sex manuals, which were written by Taoist masters,

28

masturbation in men was condemned because of this belief. These same masters were also aware that women were also capable of ejaculating, or as we commonly refer to it today, 'squirting'.

Whilst women were not specifically forbidden to masturbate, it was not a practice that was encouraged for basically the same reason as in men. Of course, we need to put this in the context of a time when women were not seen as equals in society, so their energy, or chi, was not considered to be as vital as for that of their male counterparts.

The Ancient World
Masturbation, or 'autoerotism', as it was often referred to in countries such as Ancient Greece and Egypt, was considered a very form of crude sexual expression. While masturbation was not specifically forbidden, it was frowned upon and thought to belong in the domain of prostitutes and lower-class citizens.

It was as early as 2000 BC that we began to see incidences of a disease that would plague the female species until the middle of the 20th century. 'Hysteria' in Ancient Egypt was used to describe a specific set of symptoms that included fainting, nervousness, weight loss, and depression, to name but a few. The worst symptom by far was when a woman was thought to have blood and fluid trapped in her genitals. This was also known as 'edema'. What they were talking about was basically the female equivalent of 'blue balls' in guys.

Once a diagnosis of hysteria was made, there was only one option for the poor physician. He would simply massage the patient's genitals until she orgasmed and, surprise, surprise, would receive some relief from the symptoms, all be it a temporary solution. Whilst there is no written evidence that suggests women themselves actually masturbated to help relieve the symptoms of hysteria, I think it's a pretty safe assumption that many did.

The Middle Ages

By the Middle Ages the Catholic Church was firmly established and its doctrine on masturbation was set in stone, as were most things related to sexual relations between married couples. Basically this boiled down to one thing, the only sex that was permitted was the type where the union would result in a child, or at least provided the possibility of this happening.

This was also the age where doctors became more concerned with the pollution of a person's soul if they should decide to practice masturbation. This was especially true if you happened to be a monk or a virgin or you were considered to be a high-risk patient. The treatments they offered in order to prevent this pollution ranged from simply fasting, cold baths and sitting on stones, to actually causing the affected person to punish themselves via flagellation. It's hard to determine how successful these masturbation interventions were as there is very little written evidence either way.

Eighteenth Century

As the practice of medicine and the study of anatomy became a more established practice within and during this and subsequent eras, the hype surrounding masturbation began to grow. In 1710, for example, we saw the first real book on the subject and if the title was anything to go by it was considered a very important work! *'On the heinous sin of self-pollution, and all its frightful consequences, in both sexes, considered with spiritual and physical advice to those who have already injured themselves by this abominable practice. And to seasonable admonition to the youth of the nation (of both sexes) and those whose tuition they are under, whether parents, guardians, masters or mistresses.'* I told you it was an impressive title, didn't I? This book heralded in the beginning of the modern-day campaign against masturbation that would persist well into the middle of the 20th century.

This book was by no means the only work that set out to detail the perils of masturbation or, as it was known by this time, 'onanism'. Of all these works, probably one of the most famous was written by Swiss doctor, Simmons A.A.D. Tissot and was also given a grand title: *'Onanism: – A treatise on the diseases produced by masturbation, or the dangerous effects of secret and excessive venery.'*

Tissot was the first physician to declare that the loss of the body's vital fluids via masturbation could, and would, undoubtedly cause mental illness, as well as a litany of other symptoms and was something to be avoided at all costs.

It was during the 18th century that masturbation prohibition was practiced and encouraged by physicians, parents, and the authorities with a vigor that bordered on an obsession at times, but the prohibition would not reach its peak until the 19th century, which is where we will visit next.

Nineteenth Century
During the 19th century, and especially with the reign of Queen Victoria, the feelings against the practice of masturbation reached a fever pitch. While the Victorians are well known for their puritanical views of sex, not many people realize that masturbation was now more popularly referred to as self-abuse and this was indeed how it was viewed by many of this era. Even well-known feminists of the time would warn against the nasty habits of schoolgirls, as many women believed that if you masturbated when you were younger, you would never have the ability to grow into a proper Victorian lady.

During the 19th century the medical profession began to make great strides as regards to our understanding of the way that the body actually worked. That said, it was also very much the time of what is now referred to as 'quackery'. Anyone could concoct a potion and claim it would cure just about any ill or affliction that took one's fancy. As the anti-masturbation hysteria grew many quacks and the odd doctor designed a range of devices that were intended to aid parents in their quest to stop their children from the evil and dangerous practice of 'self-pollution'.

Most of these devices were aimed at the male market, but there were a few produced with the female in mind. These, typically, would involve a chastity belt-type device or perhaps the most famous would take the form of gloves constructed of steel wool. Can you imagine sleeping with those on, let alone trying to mastur- bate? The anti- masturbation craze soon surfaced in the USA and particularly within the food market. It was a commonly held belief that eating spicy, rich food would fuel one's sexual appetite, which in turn would be hard to control. As I began to look more at the history of an entire industry that was founded in no small part on these beliefs I became more and more obsessed with the humble breakfast cereal. What follows is a quick tour around how the breakfast-cereal industry came to be in America, and the impact that anti-masturbation thoughts of the time prevailed on that industry and the entire population.

Snap, Crackle, and Porn!
Whilst most people are familiar with the humble Graham Cracker, few of us know what lead to its creation, so let me enlighten you. Sylvester Graham was a Presbyterian preacher and a free-thinker. During the 1830s the typical American diet consisted of little more than red meat and blood. From his pulpit each Sunday Graham would spend many hours highlighting the perils of poor eating and masturbation. These beliefs were based on the work of Samuel Tissot and his then-famous book: *Treatise on the Diseases Produced by Onanism.*

As influential as Tissot was on Graham's thinking, an equally strong influence came in the shape of the English clergyman, William Metcalfe, who was the first advocate of vegetarianism in America. Again Graham interpreted Metcalfe's writings and thoughts into his own, while Metcalfe argued in favor of vegetarianism on moral grounds. Graham was more concerned with the carnal passions that eating meat produced in people. At that time the stomach was considered to be the major organ in the body, so anything that inflamed it was compared to lust. Graham actively promoted a vegetarian diet and claimed it was a cure for almost every form of human sickness. The cure consisted of sexual moderation (no more than 12 times a year for a married couple), exercise (this would help with nocturnal emissions, he told us) and a proper diet.

In the 1830s Graham took his show on the road, lecturing an inquiring public about the perils of 'self-pollution'. As the first of its kind it had an amazing impact on the general populace and the man behind it was just as dynamic. He sought to revolutionize the diet and sexual behavior of an entire country and in many ways was successful. Graham knew his audience well and if he were alive today no doubt would make a wonderful spin doctor, given his grasp of rhetorical devices. He was a master at making claims that no one could disprove. Considering that he preached that masturbation caused its victims to become shy, suspicious, languid, unconcerned with hygiene and, in acute cases, to suffer from hysteria, you'll see how hard it would be for your average masturbator to disprove his theories.

Around 1834, Graham stopped lecturing about sexuality and turned his thoughts toward sound nutrition. The truth was, his lectures had become too unpopular for him to continue, but our friend Graham was determined to find a way to spread his thoughts. Graham believed that there were two kinds of hunger – sexual and nutritional – and that both kinds threatened good health.

As strange as this may seem to many of us today, the Graham movement was a powerful one back in the 1800s. By 1840, his public career was over but his ideology remained deeply ingrained in society and had influenced a number of bran-loving entrepreneurs. One of those was James Caleb Jackson (1814–1895), a diet expert who combined Graham's health-reform plan with his own ideas, which mainly consisted of hydropathy. Hydropathic therapy, also known as the 'water cure', involved applying extremely cold water – showers, tubs, soaks, and wet-packs – to different parts of the body. Jackson's real brainstorm, however, was creating a stone-like wafer out of Graham flour and water. He called his treat 'Granula' and would later go down in history as having made the first cold breakfast cereal.

Graham's legacy to the world was what we today know as the humble Graham Cracker, all be it a sweetened and processed version of the one that was served during his lifetime at the many Graham hotels and boarding houses that sprang up and catered to his devoted followers. Although Graham's career had ended, his effects on sex and nutrition teachings still remained popular and the invention by Jackson of Granula was considered a major breakthrough in medical nutrition.

Of course, back then Granula was not considered a tasty treat and was not popular at first, but Jackson, like many eminent people of the day, had an ace up his sleeve. He had a ready-made market in the form of his patients at his sanitarium in Dansville, NY, where it was served on a daily basis to the residents.

It was this sanitarium that Sister Ellen White of the Seventh Day Adventists visited and asked Jackson to duplicate his Dansville establishment in Battle Creek, Michigan, the home and world headquarters of the Seventh Day Adventist movement. This facility would later become known as the Kellogg Sanitarium, or just 'the Sans', but the fact is the institute was to play a key role in not only revolutionizing the American breakfast but also the ideas behind

34

health, nutrition, and sex.

When Sister White first opened the Sans she, too, was considered a health reformer. Inspired by Jackson and Graham, she too published a book on masturbation in 1864 called, *An Appeal to Mothers: The Great Cause of the Physical, Mental and Moral Ruin of Many of the Children of Our Time*. As we can see from the passage below, even though this text was written by a woman, women were still regarded as the weaker sex.

'Females possess less vital force than the other sex, and are deprived very much of the bracing, invigorating air, by their indoors life. The results of self-abuse in them is seen in various diseases, such as catarrh, dropsy, headache, loss of memory and sight, great weakness in the back and loins, afflictions of the spine, the head often decays inwardly. Cancerous humor, which would lay dormant in the system their lifetime, is inflamed, and commences its eating, destructive work. The mind is often utterly ruined, and insanity takes place.'

Sister White, although intelligent, proved to be no leader and the Sans floundered for about ten years until a quirky young doctor named John Harvey Kellogg took over daily operations. Kellogg was another Graham disciple and advocate. He was also highly regarded within the Adventists for his hard-hitting medical journalism. Unlike Graham, he openly embraced medical science and was constantly experimenting with wholegrain foods. Two years into the job, he invented the first Battle Creek health treat, which consisted of a mixture of oatmeal and corn meal baked into biscuits and then ground into bits.

For some reason he decided to call his treat 'Granula', a strange decision when you consider that the only other cereal on the market was also called Granula. Once they finished suing him, Kellogg took the decision to rename his new product 'Granola'. Granola wasn't the only delicacy that was served to the inmates of the Sans. Other specialties included caramel cereal coffee, Bulgarian yogurt and meat substitutes.

At one point in his career Kellogg concentrated his research solely on nuts. He wrote a paper entitled 'Nuts May Save the Race'. During this period of his studies he is believed to have invented peanut butter as well as malted nuts. As strange as it may seem now, this bland diet helped turn around the fortunes of the once-failing Sans. Kellogg believed that most of the patients admitted to the Sans simply suffered from Americanitis and the remedy was simply a change in diet. The cure rate at the Sans was remarkably high simply because no one who was seriously ill was ever admitted. Kellogg never admitted any chronic masturbators to the Sans, either. This suited his purpose and like Graham he continued to preach the doom and gloom of such abhorrent practices.

For example, on the night of his honeymoon, Kellogg spent his time writing his most famous book, *Plain Facts for Old and Young, a Warning on the Evils of Sex*. This book featured an amazing collection of symptoms and cures for the curse known as 'self-pollution' as well as covering all important sexual ills of the time, but self- pollution was by far the biggest. In this book, he included the 39 signs that would indicate to an outsider that someone in fact masturbated. The fact that this list covers just about anyone who even vaguely looks human was no accident. For example:

Sleeplessness, love of solitude, bashfulness, unnatural boldness, confusion of ideas, capricious appetite, use of tobacco, and acne.

This was a clever ploy from his point of view. Just as Graham had done before him, it was extremely difficult for anyone to prove the theories wrong. Dr Kellogg was never wrong, his way was the only way and to prove a point, although he married he never consummated his marriage to Ells Eaton and they lived in separate apartments. This was supposed to prove that sexual relationships were not necessary to obtain good health.

It's quite likely, though, that the doctor was in some way dysfunctional (one book suggests he had mumps). After break-fast every morning, he had an orderly give him an enema. This may mean he had klismaphilia, an anomaly of sexual functioning traceable to childhood in which an enema substitutes for regular sexual intercourse. For the klismaphile, putting the penis in the vagina is experienced as hard, dangerous, and repulsive work.

Whatever the reasons for his beliefs, they had long-lasting effects on society and many of the myths that still surround masturbation can be directly attributed to his way of thinking. The Sans became more and more famous and Dr Kellogg himself became something of a demagogue. He began to concentrate less on his fundamental beliefs and more on scientific facts and theories.

A major step in this direction came when a patient showed him a little wheat mattress a friend had sent her to aid her digestive problems. Invented by Henry Perky from Denver, they were what we now know as Shredded Wheat. At this time Shredded Wheat was not thought of as a breakfast food. Originally it was a main course, a natural food that followed the true Grahamite tradition. As well as the original Shredded Wheat there was a whole host of recipes associated with this biscuit. These ranged from banana croquettes with Shredded Wheat to cheese and Shredded Wheat toast – the list was endless. Perky even founded a scientific institute devoted to training demonstrators on how to educate the ordinary housewife on its uses.

In the humble Shredded Wheat the good Dr Kellogg saw the potential for the first ready-to-eat breakfast cereal and went about creating his own. After much experimentation he came up with Granose, the first flaked wheat cereal. Once again the Sans featured heavily in the development of this little wonder flake. As Kellogg put his ideas into commercial production he met with some stiff opposition, not least from Perky himself, who wasn't about to let anyone rip off his invention and had taken no less than 47 patents out with regards to Shredded Wheat. The effect of the cereal wars was that Battle Creek exploded with cereal and health-food manufacturers and almost overnight the place became known as 'cereal central'. Many more wars ensued in the battle for the cereal that would rid the world of all its ailments.

John Kellogg was finally forced to turn the ailing Kellogg's company over to his brother, William, who although he had worked at the Sans with John, had little interest in curing the public of bad eating habits and masturbation but in making money. So was born the Kellogg's brand as we now know it today, but its original founder left his legacy in the myths that still surround masturbation to this day.

Late 19th Century to early 20th Century
Remember, as far back as Ancient Egyptian times we saw the emergence of the medical but vague term 'hysteria'. At the same time as Kellogg's and Graham were busy producing cornflakes and crackers, the medical profession was busy curing women of what was thought to be the often life-threatening disease known as, you guessed it, 'hysteria'. Just as in Ancient Egypt, this disease only afflicted the female sex and caused a myriad symptoms, running the gamut from anxiety, irritability, nervousness, feelings of heaviness in the lower abdomen, sleepiness, to name but a few. Of course nowadays we recognize 'hysteria' for what it actually is: horniness.

Back then, though, the cure for hysteria was a simple one. Doctors would manually masturbate their female patients to orgasm. Of course the end results were not called 'orgasms'; instead they would be referred to as 'paroxysms'. As you can imagine, this was, in many cases, a time-consuming cure, and often a temporary one. Can you imagine how tired these doctors' hands must have been?

So, being as this was the start of the Industrial Revolution, nothing was, or at least seemed, impossible and in order to relieve their cramped hands, many doctors turned to mechanical methods to help their patients reach the desired state of paroxysm. Unfortunately these machines were often poorly constructed and caused injury to the patient, but, as is often the case, electricity came to the rescue. In 1880, more than a decade before the invention of the electric iron and vacuum cleaner, an enterprising English physician, Dr Joseph Mortimer Granville, patented the electromechanical vibrator.

The vibrator was an immediate hit with doctors and patients alike and at the turn of the century, as electricity became more widely available across American homes, the humble, if often scary by today's standards, electric vibrator became a staple in many homes. Of course, when you consider this was a time when women were still considered the 'fairer sex', the actual use for the vibrator had to be disguised. Many popular magazines of the time would sell them as 'personal massagers', although their actual use was not exactly a well-kept secret.

For a while electric vibrators were acceptable and commonplace in most American homes, but that would change with the advent of the silent movie. Silent movies were not just used to make Charlie Chaplin a superstar of his time, but also by some enterprising young men, who saw their potential to provide pornographic images. As the trade in pornography grew and images of what were considered loose, wanton women using the humble electric vibrator began to grow, the popularity of the Personal Massager became tarnished and over time vibrators all but disappeared from the American home. For now...

Late 20h Century
In spite of anti-masturbation zealots like Graham and Kellogg, masturbation was by all accounts still a popular, if secret, pastime. During the 1940s and '50s the interest in people's sexual habits began to grow, at least from a scientific and medical standpoint. The most famous of the early pioneers of American sexuality, who was not afraid to ask Americans about their sexual habits was Alfred Kinsey. His work in the '40s and '50s included studies that asked Americans what were then considered shocking questions,

such as, did they masturbate to orgasm? These studies revealed that at the time 94 per cent of American men who were asked did masturbate to orgasm, while approximately 40 per cent of American women reported that they also masturbated. Kinsey's research was, at the time, groundbreaking and in many ways opened the doors to modern-day sexual research.

In the early 1970s there was a veritable explosion in the interest surrounding America's bedroom habits. By this time we had seen the sexual revolution, women had access to the Pill and the feminist movement was gaining momentum, all of which help contribute to that interest. For example: Shere Hite surveyed 1,000,000 American women and the results were then published in a report that was known as the *Hite Report*. This was a document consisting of 510 pages that detailed the masturbation habits of the respondents. Whenever I go back and read the *Hite Report* of 1976, I'm always struck by how little attitudes to masturbation have changed since that report was done. Many of the answers to the survey mirror questions and comments I get from Clitical visitors to this day. Many women back then reported a feeling of guilt, even when they physically enjoyed the act of masturbating, and any subsequent orgasm, but we will delve into that subject a little later. What Hite did discover was this: 82 per cent of those who responded to the survey reported masturbating, so women were doing it for themselves, albeit then often feeling guilty about it.

At the same time as Hite was moving and shaking the world of female sexuality, another prominent figure was also emerging. Betty Dodson, who is now often referred to as the 'mother of masturbation'. Dodson was busy at this time extolling the benefits of masturbation, and yet her teaching encompassed so much more. Dodson would actively encourage women to embrace their vulvas and to stop thinking of them as something dirty, instead realizing that they were as unique and beautiful as their owners.

I can recall the first time I ever saw her now-famous collection of pictures that, as an artist, she had drawn. Each one depicted a real woman's vulva and highlighted beautifully that every one was different. Dobson was the first sex educator to actively promote the use of the vibrator when it came to masturbation.

During the '70s and '80s we began to see a slight change in attitudes toward masturbation in general. Whilst it was still not something that you could openly discuss with your parents, or even your friends, the shame and guilt that for so long had been a part of something that was a natural and healthy act of sexuality began to subside, at least a little.

This change in the '90s, when we once more saw something of a backlash against not just masturbation, but open sexuality in general, culminated in an incident that featured the then Surgeon General, Jocelyn Elders, who agreed that masturbation should be included in any meaningful sex education programs that were to be taught in either schools or colleges across the USA. A common misconception about that incident was that Dr Elders was condoning masturbation. She was, in fact, merely agreeing with the finding of the day as opposed to actually recommending or promoting masturbation. As a result of the media coverage of this event, President Clinton was left with little choice but to ask Dr Elders to step down from her post.

As is often the case when an incident such as the detailed one above occurs, there is a backlash. In this case that backlash took the form of one of the earlier female-friendly sex-toy stores in San Francisco, 'Good Vibrations', taking a stand. They declared that from May 1995 henceforth, May would be forever known as Masturbation Month and this is still the case at the time of writing. The mastur-bation movement was just getting underway, though, and when 'Good Vibrations', 'Babeland' and 'Grand Opening' teamed up in

41

1999, creating the very first national, Masturbation-a-Thon. The first of these events took place at San Francisco's campus theater and has, over the years, raised money for many sex-positive-based charities. In 2006, London held its first-ever live Masturbate-a-Thon, with Montreal, Canada, following suit in May 2013. All of these events have raised the profile of the much-maligned practice of masturbation and helped to shape modern-day attitudes toward masturbation.

Conclusion:

Whew, that was one journey! But as you can see from this brief and somewhat abbreviated history of masturbation, it is slowly becoming more acceptable, though there is a lot of work yet to be done before we can say it is acceptable to masturbate or, more importantly, to discuss the subject amongst our peers. It's also possible to see where many of the myths that surround self-pleasure and I figured it might be a good time to look at some of the more popular and persuasive ones that still persist.

CHAPTER 3

Masturbation Myths and Realities

According to Webster's dictionary the definition of a myth is this: 'a widely held but false belief or idea.' And, as we saw when we took our spin back in time, masturbation at various times has not just been considered as dangerous, but in some cases fatal. So if you think about it, it kind of makes sense that so many myths would have grown up around the practice. I'm pretty sure that you are familiar with many of these myths, but just in case, let's take a quick look at some of the more common ones.

You will go blind
You will grow hair on the palms of your hands
You will no longer be a virgin
It's dirty
It will stunt your growth.

Now consider this for a moment. If, according to the *Hite Report*, around 80 per cent of women choose to masturbate at some stage in their lives, the female species, as we know it, should consist of blind, hairy-palmed midgets. I think it's fair to say that I have just made my point that for the most part these myths are just that, myths, or stories told by parents to curtail their young offspring from engaging in a practice that they honestly believed would cause them real harm. These stories have persisted over generations and in many cases have taken on a life of their own.

While on the surface these myths often sound funny when applied to our modern-day lives, what they can do is lead to a great degree of guilt still being felt by a large percentage of the female population. It's also worth noting, as we discovered earlier, that the majority of these myths were directed at the guys and, to some degree, they still are. We have a tendency to forget that it has only been over the last hundred or so years that women have been seen as anywhere near equal to men and this is also true in the world of sex. Women and their sexual habits were just not as important as those of their male counterparts, and it's easy to see why much of the older sexuality texts were focused on the guys.

This is No Joke

These myths have now been swallowed, in the most part, by popular culture and, in fact, many have been turned into jokes. Masturbation has turned from something to be ashamed of to something to be ridiculed. For example: if you masturbate it's because you can't get a man. If you masturbate it's because you are ugly. If you masturbate it's because you are desperate.

These are forms of myths as well, but they are myths that have been disguised in the form of being humorous, or simply a joke, in most instances. We have even created an entire new set of words for not only masturbation itself, but most of the parts of our body that are thought of as sexual. As this book is about female masturbation, let's take a look at some of the terms that have been submitted by Clitical visitors over the years to describe the act of masturbation.

The Top Terms for Female Masturbation

Battery testing, Beat the clit, Bop, Bruise the beaver, Buff the muff, Butter the biscuit, Churn the butter, Club the clam, Clit flicking, Clit pick, Deck the nun, Dial 'o' on the pink telephone, Diddle yourself, Dig your own hole, Double-click your mouse, Feed the beaver, Feel the love, Finger bang old Mary Rotten Crotch, Finger fuck, Finger the bottle, Finger the love hole, Finger yourself, Finger your pussy, Flick the bean, Flick the flab, Flip the clit, Flip your flossy, Frigging, Get lost in the deep end, Get your fingers wet, Go knuckle deep, Jill off, Jillin', Juicin' out, Knitting, Lip Curlin', Make love juice, Mine the hole, Part the pink sea, Pat the bunny, Pat the little man in the canoe, Pedicure the camel toes, Perfume the fingers, Pet the kitty, Play piano, Play with the cat, Play the hairy banjo, Play with your remote control, Play with your yo-yo, Poke the flounder, Polish the pearl, Praise the kooter, Pump your puni, Punch Jerry Garcia in the face, Push the love button, Ride the two-finger cowboy, Rough the muff, Rub off, Rub it, Rub the button, Rub the elf, Rub the love lips, Rub the nub, Rub the pussy, Scratch the snatch, Sing in the shower, Slap the lips, Slippin' the kitten, Snuff the muff, Spank the kitty, Squeeze Mary, Squeeze the bean, Stroke the kitty, Stroke the nub, Tease the tuna taco, Tender the meat curtains, Think pink, Tickle clitty, Tickle the twat, Touch type, Touchy touch, Two-finger salute.

The one thing I think that really sticks out as you read through these names, is that none of them portray female masturbation in a good light. Several could even be described as downright distasteful, and yet they exist. The worst part is that many of these terms are used by women as a way to avoid uttering the dreaded 'M' word and I personally think that's a shame. When we disguise something by using a different term, what we do is give it new meaning. While declaring to your friends that you are off to polish your pearl, or flick your bean, what you are actually saying is, 'I masturbate, but I'm still too embarrassed to use the proper word, instead I prefer to dress it up in a neat, tidy package, or as an inside joke.'

A funny thing happened when I began writing this book. I was forced to tell people that I had a book contract, which, in turn, forced me to answer the inevitable question, 'That's awesome! What's the book about?' I could have taken the easy path and simply lied. Instead I chose to tell them simply that it was about female masturbation. Then would come the awkward silence as people digested what I had just said, then came the reactions. These ranged from, 'That's nice' to 'Oh my gosh, I want a copy when you've finished it' to 'Really, why would you write about "that"?' I ran the entire gamut, but I don't like to lie to people, either. This is what I do and this is what I choose to write about. In all good faith, I could hardly sit here and type about how you should masturbate and not be ashamed and then hide behind a lie when it came to tell people the truth about what I was writing.

The more I've opened up and told people what I'm writing about the more interested people have become. At first I figured everyone would consider it a joke, but to my surprise people have been nothing but supportive and I'm willing to bet that if you could find the courage to tell at least your closest friend that you masturbate and actually use the correct word, you will be surprised by the outcome as well. I'm not suggesting you should stand on the roof of your building and shout that you masturbate, but until we learn to open up about the subject and use the correct word, masturbation will likely always be thought of as partner sex's ugly sister and I, for one, think that's a shame. I hope after reading this you'll agree.

To Masturbate or Not, That is the Question?

Now we've put many of the popular masturbation myths to bed, so to speak, maybe it's time to turn our attention to whether you should or should not masturbate. More than this, though, I want you to examine the reasons why you might choose not to when scientific evidence overwhelmingly tells us that masturbation is a healthy and safe practice.

Now, before you start sending me angry emails and letters, I'm in no way saying that anyone, including you, MUST masturbate. Like everything else in life it is a personal choice and all I'm asking you to do is to take a few minutes out of your life to examine why you actively choose not to do something. Over the years I've been running Clitical I've collected a pretty comprehensive list of reasons why one might choose to masturbate, and the benefits of doing so. Again, let me stress that I am not telling you that you MUST masturbate, but it would be remiss of me not to list the many benefits that could be achieved by doing so. (Okay, I admit that many of these are funny, but they are still relevant).

80 Reasons to Masturbate

Everybody else is doing it.

It helps you become more comfortable with your body.

You will get a better idea of what pleases you, something you can share with a lover later.

You won't be as irritable at work or school.

You can develop control and staying power in a low-stress situation.

You can discover that many areas of your body are sensitive and excitable other than your genitals.

You're trying to quit smoking and you have to do something with your hands.

You feel the need to tap off excess fluid on occasion to keep your body running at optimal efficiency.

You have always wanted to create a world record, so you need to practice.

Look at this body! Who wouldn't want to touch it?

47

It's safe sex, as long as you watch your aim.

You can't sleep.

There's never anything good on TV.

You just wanted to make sure everything was still in good working order.

Because every time you do, an angel spasms.

Exercises the wrist and reduces the chance for carpal tunnel syndrome.

It's mine and I can wash it as fast as I want, okay?

It's really, really difficult to get pregnant when you're the only one there.

Even if you do have company, it's not easy to get pregnant if you're careful.

You can stay a virgin for years without getting twitchy.

It helps to maintain good pelvic blood flow and strong PC muscles.

Big money-saver on dinner and alcohol.

It reduces menstrual cramps.

Men who stimulate their prostate glands during masturbation reduce their incidence of prostate infections.

It stimulates your creativity and enriches your fantasy life.

You're asserting your independence!

You don't have to depend on anyone but yourself for your orgasms.

You can get it any time you want.

You can do anything you want without having to explain it to a bewildered partner.

You're helping to establish the philosophy that sex is good in, by, and for itself; and that there is nothing whatever wrong about experiencing it as a fine thing in its own right.

It's cheaper than Zoloft and the side effects are better.

The love of your life is currently unavailable

The love of your life is currently available, but isn't interested right now.

The love of your life is currently available, but likes watching you.

It releases endorphins into the bloodstream, and that's good for you.

Eases the strain and anxiety of long traffic jams.

Reduces the need to ask for sex during times when it might be inconvenient or unwanted, like when you're piloting your new jet aircraft.

It keeps you from hitting all the people who really need hitting.

Because you always call the next day.

No scrambling for birth control.

Better than nagging your partner for sex, and they might just join in.

You'll be able to grip your golf club with more confidence.

You can join the Mile-High Club without trying to cram two people in that little bathroom.

In 1972 the American Medical Association declared masturbation a normal sexual activity, and you're celebrating.

You can take all the time you need.

You're doing your part as an American to keep the sex-toy economy thriving.

Because the son of a bitch popped and went to sleep on you.

Your next-door neighbor has been watching you through the window and you think it's time to take the relationship to the next level.

Keeping one hand under the table at all times is a valuable defensive pose. Well that's what a friend once told me.

Helps improve your backhand.

Because you can't reach with your mouth.

You paid for your dinner and the movie, so you're probably required to.

You're watching an adult movie and there is an implied contract between you and the movie's stars.

To glorify God and His creations.

49

You don't have to count days first.

It's performance art.

Because it makes your website membership spike every time you do it.

Flipping burgers only takes one hand, so…

Because no one else is good enough for you. You barely qualify.

The cast came off today.

It's non-carcinogenic, non-fattening, and low in sodium.

Because you are entitled to life, liberty, and the pursuit of happiness, and all three are just within reach right now.

clitical@yahoo.com told you to.

It doesn't require equipment (although there's quite a large industry ready to supply you if you want some).

You said too many Hail Marys, and you simply have to even it out.

Because this isn't just a casual fling – you really love yourself.

It was integral to the plot.

You've got a lot of love to give.

You needed new material for your 'Best Of' DVD.

Helps keep you warm on cold nights.

It's what the 'pause' button was invented for.

You've heard that if you don't use parts of your body they atrophy and drop off, and that's scary.

It's part of your low-impact aerobic full-body workout. Ten reps, pause, repeat as needed.

You brought one too many cucumbers for dinner and waste is a sin.

Because (drum roll) it's there.

Because it's FREE.

What else are you supposed to do during commercial breaks?

If you want it done right you have to do it yourself.

You're ambidextrous so you get two for the price of one.

It feels good.

All joking aside, female masturbation has plenty of proven scientific benefits, and as we can see from the list, some that are not so scientific. One of the biggest benefits is that it allows you a safe place to become more comfortable with your own curves, folds, and sexual anatomy. When I say 'safe' I mean this in a couple of different senses. It's really, really difficult to get pregnant or catch a STD when you are the only one in the room. The only exception to that is if you bring a toy, whether homemade or purchased, into your masturbation routine and we will look at the risks and precautions you can take in a later chapter and you still can't get pregnant on your own!

The other way in which I mean 'safe' is that you are within your own environment as opposed to another person's. You can explore your own body without fear of judgment, condemnation, or ridicule. You get to choose the pace at which you progress with your learning, unlike when you are with a partner, who may or may not be more knowledgeable in the sexual arena than you are.

Another huge benefit is that like any sex act, masturbation has the ability to allow your body to de-stress. What happens when you masturbate? You reduce stress, boost your immune system, make yourself more comfortable and relaxed, and send endorphins into your bloodstream, which make you happier. The chemicals released during any sexual activity boost your mood, elevate your happiness, and feelings of wellbeing and contentment.

When you masturbate to orgasm, you don't just feel good for those few seconds; you're genetically hotwired for a reward. You're going to feel good for the rest of the day or night – a side effect of masturbation, for many women, is it helps them sleep.

Conclusion:

Hopefully, after reading this you have a good sense of where and why the most popular of the masturbation myths came from. Most of these myths were established in a time before scientific research was available. Of course, we still have a lot to discover when it comes to female sexuality and especially female masturbation. I hope that you are now agreeing with me that the benefits of masturbation far outweigh the downsides. Actually, I'm wondering if there are any actual downsides to masturbation, but we will leave that for a later chapter. Right now, let's take a look at some of the ways in which we can overcome some of the moral objections that you may have to the ancient art of masturbation, shall we?

CHAPTER 4

Morals, Guilt, and Salvation

So I can sit here and write about all the benefits that masturbation can afford you as a woman until I'm blue in the face, but the truth is, unless you believe that masturbation is truly good for you, we are likely both wasting our time. So let's spend some time discovering why you might have, what I like to refer to as, a psychological block when it comes to masturbation.

Don't Touch Your Privates
One of the main reasons that many women have a psychological block when it comes to masturbation, is the fact that we are told from an early age that our privates are, well, our privates. They are tucked between our thighs and there they stay and are supposed to stay untouched until the magical Prince Charming comes along and then we open them and the world of sexuality will blossom under the careful tutelage of said prince. Yes, it's a fairy tale, but it's a very pervasive fairy tale when you think about it. Holy hell! Walt Disney built an empire on the 'prince will come and save you' fairy tale.

Boys are more often than not taught not to touch their own privates in public or in the living room but to reserve that kind of activity to the confines of their own bedrooms. Girls are often not afforded even that little bit of advice, instead being told that their privates should never be touched, period. At least until they fall in love with the handsome prince who will free them from the shackles of sexual lust.

Whilst penises are given names such as 'willy' and 'dick', girls' bits and pieces are often referred to as 'fish', 'meat', and 'curtains' and an entire litany of words that should never be used to describe something that is designed to do nothing but give you pleasure. Yet the names persist and they more often than not have a negative impact on the way we view our genitals. Who in their right mind wants to touch a wet fish, after all?

God forbid that as a female you get caught by a parent engaging in masturbation when you are young. You will likely be told that your fish is a special place that should only be touched once you fall in love and are married. It's a sacred place and a very private one. Oftentimes this will be the extent of any conversation that you might have on the subject of masturbation, but the one thing you will take away from these conversations and names is a negative one. Your private parts are private, touching them is something that only 'dirty' girls do, and you're bad for enjoying any pleasure you might get from touching your private parts.

As we discussed in chapter three the reasons for these negative connotations are many and varied, but are complete myths. The truth is you own your private parts and if you choose to touch them, who is anyone else to tell you that you shouldn't? Unfortunately, the overwhelming negative messages we receive about our bodies when we are younger are often easier to think about than to overcome. The good thing is that with some work on your part it is possible to overcome them and learn to enjoy your own private parts and discover your sexual self.

Creating a Positive Image
In many cases it's far easier to believe that we are bad or unattractive than we are good or beautiful and when it comes to masturbation and the ability to orgasm this can have some serious negative effects. The exercises that I suggested in chapter one were designed to not only help you realize that your entire body is part of your sexual being, but your self image is an important part of the solo sex puzzle.

There are few ladies in the world who haven't at some stage in their life felt the impact of a negative self-image. It's easy to find yourself caught up in a cycle of negativity, and it's something that you should be aware of. As females we are constantly bombarded with images and messages telling us what we should look like, how we should act, and who we should aspire to be like. It's hard to compete with many of these images and messages, but it's worth remembering that these images are not your reality. No one else lives in your body, no one else is like you, looks like you, or acts like you.

The simple truth is the way in which you view your body will have an effect on how the rest of the world views you. Learning to love the skin that you will live in for the rest of your life is a great start when it comes to a positive self-image.

I believe that we all have one part of our body that we at least like. For me this is my arms. They are strong, they hold the things I love, and I kinda like the way they look. I challenge you to select one part of your own body that you already either like or love, and start by focusing on the reasons why you like it. Once you have figured out all the good things that one part of

55

your body can do and why you like it, begin to work on other parts of your body. It's surprising how differently you can see your own body if you focus on what your body does for you and what an amazing piece of machinery it really is rather than focusing on the negative parts.

One of the great things about masturbation is that it is a low-pressure sex act in many ways. As you are the only one there, no one but yourself is going to judge you. The only trouble is that often women are their own worst critics and this can impact both your solo and partnered sexual experiences. By allowing yourself the freedom to explore your own body through masturbation, or simply touching, you can learn to not only appreciate your own body, but also become more comfortable with both sex and yourself.

Out in the Open
As we've seen in other chapters, many of us will have masturbated in secrecy over the years. For me, masturbation was an activity that was carried out under cover of darkness, and more often than not under the covers, for many years. I'm sure this is true of a lot of women. What this did was subconsciously teach me that masturbation was something I should feel guilty about, but more than that, the sexual part of my being was something that should remain in the shadows.

One of the reasons I love to masturbate in front of a mirror or film myself now is that it's an open act of defiance against those guilt-ridden sessions, which were in retrospect very negative. Of course, I'm not saying that it's appropriate to simply take your clothes off in the middle of the public library and start masturbating. What I am saying is it's okay to bring mastur-bation out from under the cover of darkness (or at least the bed covers).

Religious Masturbation

One of the biggest reasons that many women experience guilt when it comes to masturbation is religion. Again, before you get angry with me, I want to be clear. I am in no way, shape, or form condemning anyone's religious beliefs here or those of their parents. What I am saying is that oftentimes, religious belief of both our parents, and as we become adults, ourselves, can shape our thoughts and actions when it comes to masturbation.

Like everything else in life, choosing to masturbate is just that, a choice, and a very personal one. I would never tell someone what they should or shouldn't do and especially if doing that something goes against someone's beliefs. What I am trying to say is that there is nothing wrong with challenging or checking the facts that surround your own religious beliefs and masturbation. Oftentimes, these beliefs are not founded on whichever book or god you chose to worship, but over time have grown from a period in history when humans had less understanding of sexuality, and this can be especially true for women and sexuality.

Conclusion:

There are as many reasons to feel guilty as there are ways to masturbate. Learning to love yourself for who you are is just one step on the road to overcoming any guilt you might feel for masturbating, but it's about much more than that. It's about learning to love the sexual side of yourself for who you are, no matter what your religion, creed, color, or race. It's about accepting that for all your faults and problems, there is only one of you and you have to make the best of what you have. By learning to be comfortable in your own skin and touching your own body without shame, you are on the way to being a better you, and who doesn't want that?

CHAPTER 5

Orgasms: It's About the Journey, Not the Destination

When we masturbate, the goal is generally to experience the some-times seemingly elusive, earth-shattering orgasm. Over the years two of the questions I've been asked the most at Clitical is what does an orgasm feel like, and when will I know if I've had one?

The trouble with the first question is that there is actually no definitive way an orgasm feels, for each person and each experience it's different. The only true answer to the second part of that question is, you **WILL** know when you experience one. As I said before, I wasn't even sure what I was experiencing in my teenage years. I just knew it felt good and I wanted to do it more.

Sometimes I feel too much information can have the opposite effect to what is intended. Let me explain a little more. There was a time when simply achieving orgasm was enough. Those of us in the orgasm club knew that we had made ourselves feel good, but we didn't always know what the correct word for the experience was. But it didn't matter. All that mattered was that it felt good, not what it was called. Then came the explosion of orgasm literature. *Cosmopolitan* and *Redbook* spent hours telling their readers that they had every right to expect an orgasm, either from solo or partnered sex and over time the message somehow came down to the fact that if you didn't experience one you were either missing out or were doing sex all wrong. The other downside was that if your partner wasn't capable of giving you an orgasm, they were basically not good in the sack and didn't deserve your attention. For so long communication was something that was put on the back burner when it came to any sexual experience, with the only thought or goal being the pot at the end of the rainbow: an orgasm.

Over time, this message was again distorted by the media and society at large and women were told it was their birthright to have an orgasm. Now don't get me wrong. I'm not saying that having an orgasm is not a great thing, but we became a society that to some degree was orgasm-obsessed. The only thing that suddenly mattered when it came to sex was that a woman experienced an orgasm. While that sounds great, the reality was that there were many women who still have never experienced an orgasm that have been left out of the orgasm conversation.

The other downside of making sex so goal-orientated was that we became so focused in the end result we all forgot about the journey. I want you to consider this for a few minutes if you will:

You are embarking on a long car journey; one that you have been looking forward to. You pack all the things that you feel you will need during the trip and when you finally arrive at your destination. You start off with a lot of anticipation, but even as excited as you might be by the thought of reaching your destination it does not stop you looking out of the window on the journey, or perhaps stopping to take in a sight or two that also interests you. Yet when it comes to sex, so many times I read of people being so focused on achieving orgasm that they miss the nuances often involved in the getting there. As we saw in chapter one, and especially if you tried any of the exercises, there is so much more your body is capable of sexually than simply giving you an orgasm, and I personally believe that if you go straight for the orgasm, you are likely missing out on other things that can bring you pleasure.

Relax Just Do It!
Anxiety is the orgasm's biggest enemy and one of the reasons I believe that we have to make any sexual experience focused on the journey as opposed to the destination. Despite the fact that an orgasm is, in fact, one of the most simple pleasures in life, it sure can generate a lot of anxiety: probably more than any other single topic when it comes to sexuality. Questions like: Am I taking too long to orgasm? Is my orgasm strong enough? What type of orgasm did I just have? became commonplace in advice columns, where once the only real question was: How do I know if I've orgasmed?

The human mind is a complex and strange instrument, but a very powerful one and it has a weird habit of playing tricks on its owner at times. Just when we think we know ourselves well sexually, our brains can throw in a roadblock. Our usual five minutes to orgasm take ten, we might suddenly no longer be able to achieve an orgasm period, or we lose our sex drive altogether.

Fake it Till You Make it
I'll let you into a secret, when I was younger and began my journey into partnered sex, I was so worried that it was taking me too long to orgasm when I was with my partner, and they were gonna get bored with me. So, like a lot of women of the time, I faked an orgasm or two. Looking back, it was crazy, but it was easier than worrying about what they might think. Nowadays I fake nothing. If it takes me 20 minutes to get there, so be it. What changed my

60

opinion, you might well ask?

In a word: masturbation. I learned more about my own body and orgasms through masturbation than any other part of my sexual world. I realized that whilst a partner could give me an orgasm, I first needed to give myself permission to have one. I also knew how my body responded to certain touches because I had spent time exploring my body via masturbation. I know that I need lots of clitoral stimulation in order to achieve an orgasm, but I also know that once I have achieved one clitoral orgasm I can actually then achieve an orgasm simply from thrusting a dildo into me. The information that I have learned about my own body when I am playing solo have often translated into a more satisfying part-nered experience, simply because I already know this information.

Can I Have More Please?
Yes, Virginia, it's true, women have one advantage over men when it comes to the orgasm train, in that we are capable of achieving multiple orgasms. Our male counterparts are often limited to one orgasm, although this is not always true, but in general men, require a greater recovery time between orgasms than women. Whether you view this as a curse or a blessing is a very much a personal preference. The thing that I want to point out is that just because you can have multiple orgasms, there is no rule that says you have to have them – or even that you should. Sometimes one is simply enough to satisfy your sexual hunger and at other times no amount can satisfy you.

If you do decide that you want to try for multiple orgasms, there are three basic rules you should follow:

Back off, breathe, and move. Once you have experienced your first orgasm, you may well find your clitoris is too sensitive to touch, and this is where the back-off rule comes in. If you find your clitoris is too sensitive to touch, simply swap the method of stimulation. For example: if you were using a vibe, try using your fingertips instead and tread lightly, so to speak. This is when rules two and three should be combined. As you touch yourself, take deep panting breaths and rock your pelvis in time with your breathing. What you are doing is giving your clitoris time to readjust and to build some sexual tension back into your body. After a few minutes, the feelings will hopefully turn from painfully sensitive to wonderfully pleasurable. There are some women who claim that the more they orgasm the more intense the feelings become, whilst others find their orgasms become less intense the more they experience. The simple truth is, you will never know unless you try!

The Right Type of Orgasm
There was a time when simply achieving an orgasm was great news and for many women signaled that they were 'normal', but as knowledge and interest grew around sexuality, a simple orgasm would no longer suffice, it seemed. Now it was not good enough to simply achieve an orgasm, we were supposed to be able to identify the type of orgasm that we had just experienced. Only being able to have a clitoral orgasm was no longer enough. Now we had a whole pantheon of orgasm types that we had to try and obtain. In other words, we inadvertently created the orgasm Olympics. Instead of just being happy to orgasm, we were supposed to examine the type of orgasm we had just experienced. Had I just experienced a new type of orgasm, or was it, in fact, the same type but just a little stronger, and if so, why? It took me a while to realize just how silly this was, but once I did and stopped worrying about the type of orgasm I had achieved, I began to relax and simply enjoy the sensations and the aftereffects of any orgasm I did achieve.

Even today there is a lot of argument in the scientific community about the types of orgasm women are really capable of achieving. I've seen and read about as many as 11 types of orgasms that women are thought to be capable of achieving, but I think it's easy to get caught up in the 'my orgasm is better than your orgasm game', and is not something that I personally prescribe to. So for this book I decided to keep things simple, in that there are basically three recognized types of orgasm: clitoral, vaginal, and blended. So let's take a closer look at the two types and what they can mean to you sexually.

Clitoral Orgasms
Clitoral orgasm, as the name suggests, is one that comes from direct stimulation of the clitoris. If you recall, we discovered earlier that this little hot button of desire has only one purpose in life: to give you pleasure. That's not to say the clitoris is like the genie in the lamp and all you have to do is rub it and all your orgasm wishes will come true. Oftentimes this is far from the case, and often it takes a combination of many things in order to release the potential pleasure that your clit is capable of giving you.

Your clitoris did not come with an instruction manual and if you think of this as a disadvantage you might want to rethink that. If all clitorises were created equally then sex solo or partnered would not be anywhere near as much fun as it could be. Experimentation is the only way you can really find what works for you and the best way to rub, tap, or poke that genie into life.

Often, just as solo sex has been seen as partnered sex's ugly sister, the clitoral orgasm is often seen as the least-desired of the three main types of orgasm. This is, in part, because a clitoral orgasm is generally the easiest of the three types to obtain or reach. It does NOT mean that this is any less of an intense orgasm for many women. Nor does it make you less of a woman if it's the only type you find you are able to reach. It means simply that your body is designed for clitoral orgasms and that is something that should, in my opinion, be celebrated.

Vaginal Orgasms

A vaginal orgasm is simply an orgasm achieved by inserting something into your vagina. This could be your fingers, a sex toy, or a penis. Back in the early 20th century a well-known psychologist, Sigmund Freud, declared that a woman who had a vaginal orgasm was to be considered mature, compared to a woman who only orgasmed via clitoral stimulation. Thanks in part to Freud's assumptions, vaginal orgasms are often thought of as a superior type of orgasm, but the truth is they are almost as rare as unicorns. There are few women in the world who can orgasm just by thrusting an object into the vagina. Of course, we have to put Freud's observations into context here and understand that his observations were based not on any study of the female anatomy, but on the fact that women at the turn of the 20th century were still very much thought of as inferior to men, especially sexually. So it would make sense that Freud might make the assumption that a woman who could orgasm via a thrusting motion (a penis) might be more mature. Today, of course, this has little bearing on a woman's ability to orgasm, other than the psychological effects of this myth.

G-Spot Anyone?

You've likely heard of the almost infamous g-spot by now, and this is generally located at the front of your vaginal wall, and can, with the right stimulation, provide you with a great orgasm. The downside of a g-spot orgasm is that initially it can produce a feeling that mimics needing to pee urgently. For a number of women this can be a very uncomfortable feeling, and often stops them from achieving a g-spot orgasm as they stop before the feeling subsides. If you feel this urge and you have already emptied your bladder prior to masturbating, if you can work through this feeling the orgasm that might well ensue is often spectacular.

Finding the Elusive G-Spot

The actual location of the g-spot varies from woman to woman, with some having theirs closer to the entrance of the vagina and others farther back, but just follow this technique and you can't go wrong. It is best to do this in a highly aroused state. It can be difficult to find when not aroused, as it is usually a small area that becomes quite enlarged during arousal. Take a lubed finger, whichever one is most comfortable. Turn your palm up. Now insert the finger barely inside the vagina, remaining on its 'ceiling'. Now, very slowly, move the finger deeper into the vagina, being sure to stay against the ceiling. You will soon find the pubic bone. You can't miss it. Once you find the pubic bone, move back just a little bit farther. Again, be sure to stay on the ceiling. Move just behind the pubic bone and feel around for a small area about the size of a bean, or so. It has a different texture than the surrounding area. I like to describe the texture as being similar to corduroy, as it feels like it has ridges. I have also heard it described as feeling spongy. That will be the g-spot.

It is worth noting here that whilst the g-spot can be a wonderful extension of your orgasm play, not everyone enjoys having it stimulated. In fact, for some women it can be a turn-off rather than a turn-on to have it stimulated this way. That said, as always, the only way to discover if it works for you is to locate it and try it. There is a new breed of sex toy on the market designed to help you discover this hidden spot and it can make the task easier.

Blended Orgasms

As the name suggests, these are orgasms that are achieved by blending the two types described above. The truth is that most orgasms are blended in some way or another. Remember I told you that the clitoris was more like an iceberg than a button? (If not, go back and read chapter one while I think of a suitable punishment.) Your clitoris is the visible part of that iceberg, but it extends a lot deeper into your vagina and that is what you're stimulating when you are trying to achieve any kind of orgasm that involves penetration. By using a mixture of clitoral and thrusting stimulation it's possible to master the blended orgasm. Many women report that these types of orgasm are extremely intense.

Conclusion:

There is still so much we don't understand about female sexuality and especially orgasms. The truth is, each and every orgasm you will likely experience throughout your life will be as unique and individual as you are. This is one of the reasons I believe that masturbation is so important when it comes to creating a strong foundation to your sexual house. It's also one of the main reasons that I think rather than obsessing over which type of orgasm you have just experienced it's a lot more important to lie back, relax, and simply enjoy them. I'm not sure about you, but I prefer to let the scientists fight about that topic because life is simply too short as it is.

CHAPTER 6

Mind Over Matter

The biggest sex organ you possess is, in fact, your brain. Think about it for a second. Without your brain, it makes no odds what you do with your hands, as it will have no effect. Good sex, especially solo sex can (and probably should) begin mentally long before it turns physical. Is it possible to turn yourself on simply by going through the mechanics of sex, such as: playing with yourself physically, but let's face it's so much easier when you are turned on or in the mood before you begin. How you get turned on is as individual as your fingerprints, but there are some shortcuts that in general will work for many. So let's start by taking a look at how our mind can influence our hands and turn us onto a good solo sex session.

Give Yourself Permission

Of all the messages you take from this book, I hope that this is the one you will take to heart. Your mind and body are, as we have discussed before, not separate things. One cannot function without the other. Think about this for a second. If I cut off your arm you could still use your brain, but if I cut off your head we are looking at a completely different scenario. Don't worry! I'm not about to ask you to cut off your head, or your arm, for that matter. What I am trying to do is to make you realize that unless you use your mind to give your body permission to do something, it's likely your body will not respond, or at the very least not respond in the way you would like it to.

Females have an amazing tendency to put their own needs, sexual or otherwise, on the bottom of any want list they may have. This is especially true if you have a partner and a couple of kids to consider. Giving yourself permission to take time out and simply enjoy your own body can often seem like a selfish act. If you do choose to take that time, but your head is filled with thoughts of tomorrow's work schedule, what the kids are having for lunch, or any other manner of flotsam that is apt to creep into your thoughts at the wrong time, it's hard to allow your mind to just feel what your body is trying to tell it.

I think this is especially true when it comes to solo sex. When you have a partner, it's much easier to be present in the moment as you have a kind of solidarity with your partner. They are also taking time out of their busy schedule to spend time with you. When you are on your lonesome, it's easy to let other things take priority, and, to be honest, when you do that you are doing yourself something of a disservice. Unless you first give yourself permission to enjoy some alone time, and, more importantly, participate fully in the experience, you are unlikely to get as much out of the experience as you could.

Understanding that you are as worthy of your time as anyone else on the long list that you likely have is an important step in learning to enjoy solo sex time.

Fantasies Are Us

There as many fantasies in this world as your mind can create and the great thing about creating fantasies is you can go anywhere you want, be with anyone you want, and do anything that takes your fancy and all in the privacy of your own head. It doesn't get much better than that, now, does it? No one to tell you what's right or wrong? Well, except you, and occasionally, I will admit, that can be a problem, but we will look at that a little later.

The great thing about sexual fantasies is they offer you a safe way to explore what may turn you on. No one says you ever have to act on a particular fantasy that might turn you on, and in many cases doing so would be either impractical or might even get you arrested: the type of fantasies that are considered taboo by society at large, but as long as they stay in your head there is nothing wrong with them. The only time I would advise you to get help with a fantasy is if it becomes more of a fetish than a fantasy. In other words, the only way that you can obtain an orgasm is by thinking or acting on the particular fantasy that turns you on. If you ever find this to be the case, my best advice would be to find a good sex therapist.

Many women, myself included, find that they have specific scenes or scenarios that they will use when they masturbate. Over the years I've come to view my fantasies as just another sex toy. The great thing about these types of sex toys is that they cost me nothing, and they belong only to me, unless of course I feel comfortable enough with my partner to share them.

The one thing that fantasies are excellent for is to help you mentally get in the mood for the physical effects of masturbation. Most women are familiar with the effect that thinking 'dirty', as it's often called, will have on their vulvas and oftentimes their breasts. You know that time when you thought about the hot guy that works in the office with you, the one you suddenly found yourself imagining throwing you over the desk and doing all manner of things to you? Try and recall the physical response your body had just to that stream of thought and it's easy to see how powerful fantasies can be.

As I said before, there are certain scenarios and fantasies that have become as familiar to me as my favorite teacup. Does that mean that over the years those fantasies have always stayed the same? No, but I have found that they almost always had a recurring theme within then. By taking the time to look at what turns you on mentally, it's possible to increase your enjoyment and understanding of masturbation, and ultimately your orgasms, and we all want to be the mistress of our own orgasms, even if we are with a partner.

As I stated before, fantasies come in all shapes and sizes. There are no right or wrong fantasies as they are of your own creation. Whilst in the real-world sense they may be deemed 'wrong' – that is only if you were to choose to act on them – for the most part they are harmless as long as they stay in your head. So let's take a look at some of the more common fantasies, and some of the less common, for starters. Who knows, you might find yourself a new one here as well. Note: these are in no particular order of popularity:

1: Professional Fantasies
These types of fantasies include the ever-popular: doctor and nurse, school teacher and student, cop and prisoner, lawyer and client, boss and coworker, bar man and drinker, to mention but a few of the professional situations that feature amongst many fantasies. Of course there are many more, and the good thing is they are all limited only by the imagination of the person fantasizing.

2: Threesomes, Foursomes, and Moresomes

This type of fantasy should be pretty self-explanatory, but just in case it's not, these fantasies simply involve at least three people, including yourself. The combinations and situations within this popular fantasy are limitless. You could, for example, be having sex with your partner as well as your best friend at the same time.

3: Sex With Someone Other Than Your Partner

This could be grouped with fantasy number two, but I think it deserves its own category. This is mainly because threesomes, foursomes, and moresomes fantasies will often include your current partner. The type of fantasy I'm talking about here is one that specifically excludes your current partner.

For example, many women enjoy the idea of sex with another woman, and if the sexual fantasies section at clitical.com is anything to go by, this is also a very popular theme when masturbating.

4: Stranger Danger/Public Sex

Public sex is all about creating dangerous situations and, for the most part, are not things that you would ever think of acting out in real life. That's not to say that you shouldn't, but it does come with the caveat of being aware of, and having knowledge of, the laws where you live. The idea of having sex in a public place can be a very alluring thought for many women.

The stranger/danger or rape fantasy can be a tricky one for a lot of women. It is a fantasy that in no way, shape, or form means that you actually want to be raped. It's simply an idea that turns you on, and that is something to remember when it comes to all fantasies.

5: Star-Struck Fantasies

These are also known as 'celebrity worship fantasies' and are more

71

popular than you might imagine. As an example, if the thought of Justin Timberlake lying in your bed and pleasing you for an entire night floats your boat, then go with the flow. These types of fantasies have the advantage of being as large as the personalities that feature within the fantasy. Most celebrities are rich, and so the sky is the limit as regards when and where. As always, all that limits you is your imagination.

6: Bondage/Discipline Fantasies

Many women enjoy the idea of playing with submission and domination in their own heads. You could be the dominatrix whose willing slave follows your every command to the letter. Conversely you could be the willing slave who chooses to follow her master. Remember it's your head and you can be anything you want to be and no one else has to ever know.

7: Taboo Fantasies

Society has put constraints on what is socially acceptable when it comes to sex, but as yet there are no plans to implement the thought police that I am aware of. Some sexual taboos include sex with animals, kids, and non-consensual sex. There are laws against these three top taboos, and with good reason, but sometimes it's the very fact that they are taboo that can make them such a powerful turn-on.

These are just a few ideas for fantasies that you may, or may not, choose to explore in the safety of your own head. You can also pull fantasy ideas from popular mainstream movies, books, and especially, erotica. The only thing that really limits you here is, well, yourself. Try letting go and allowing your imagination to go where it wants as you touch yourself. If you need a starting point, why not pull from your memories, or use the image of that hot guy/woman you met at the coffee shop this morning. Remember, no one but you knows what you are thinking, after all.

Porn, Porn, and More Porn

There are plenty of women who will tell you that mainstream, conventional porn does nothing for them and, in some cases, will turn them off. The trick I found with porn is to take it for what it is rather than what I thought it should be.

While it's true that the majority of visual porn is made with guys in mind, there is some porn that is made for women by women. Probably the most famous female porn purveyor is Candida Royalle, and at the time she made films such as *One Size Fits All*, they were revolutionary and unlike many of the scenes in conventional porn. It was not just about the guy or the money shot, it was about the plot, characters, and the viewer in general. Before you say you can't stand porn, you might want to check out some of her films.

The great thing about watching porn by yourself is that there is no judge or jury, as it often seems to be when we watch it with others. By allowing yourself to just enjoy the images rather than look at them with a critical eye, you can often find things that do turn you on. Be warned, though, oftentimes you can be surprised by the scenes that turn you on. It is also worth remembering and mentioning, also, that porn is merely fantasy fodder. It's not meant to represent reality, despite what you may have been told. I've been around a long time and I've yet to go to bed with six-inch stilettos on, for example, but if you watch a lot of porn, you might think that this was a normal thing that everyone who has sex is doing. Think of it as sexual sci-fi, if you like. Yes, the people on the screen are real people, but just like Dr Who they are merely actors playing out someone else's fantasy. Someone wrote the script that plays out in front of your eyes, and someone else is directing it and playing in it.

Fast Forward and Pause Are Your Friends

When it comes to porn there is one thing that many of us forget; we are in control of what we watch. I like to choose a film with many scenes that fit within my favorite fantasies. For me, this might mean I choose a film that has a variety of shorter scenes that all fit under the bigger umbrella of the actual fantasy of threesomes. I will then start to watch each scene, and I can almost guarantee that there are always one or two scenes that each time I watch that movie I will come back to, because, quite simply, they are the ones that turn me on. You can try the same thing to at least get your juices flowing and then you can take things into your own hands from there.

The Softer Side of Porn

Porn does not have to be full-on, in-your-face sex for the sake of sex. Many women will watch soft-core porn that leaves something, and in some cases, a lot, to the imagination. If you've ever watched programming that is referred to as 'adult' on cable, the stuff that is on after 12:00 pm, you will be familiar with soft-core porn. You will see only breasts and bums in this genre, but they can be just as hot as any full- blown, show-me-everything hardcore porn. Soft-core movies give your brain enough information to process the image and allow it to fill in the blanks. Over the years, soft-core porn has spawned quite a few of my own personal favorite fantasy scenarios and are worth taking a look at.

Mainstream Movies

There is fantasy fodder a-plenty to be found in mainstream movies. It's just a question of thinking about the plot and the main characters and using your own imagination to fill in the blanks, so to speak. For example: the film *Pretty Woman* is filled with sexy possibilities, and although the script writer chose not to take the plot in that direction, it doesn't mean you can't in the privacy of your own head.

Book Me In

Unless you have been living under a stone, it's unlikely that you have escaped the hype and fuss that is *Fifty Shades of Grey*. No matter what you may have thought of the book and Ms James's writing, the one thing that this book has achieved has been to bring erotica from the back shelf of independent book stores and put it up front and center of many a mainstream book store. In my opinion this can never be a bad thing and has opened up many conversations about erotica as both a genre and a way to turn yourself on.

Before *Fifty Shades*, erotica was something that, like masturbation, you did under the cover of darkness, in the privacy of your own home or room. Now, with the advent of e-readers, it's a lot easier to read erotica in the coffee shop, on the bus, or even at work on break. Psttt, it's also a lot sexier...

Aural Sex

Audio books are one of the fastest-growing mediums out there and the good news is that plenty of erotic titles and anthologies have taken to the aural form of communication. Whilst you might feel that you don't have the time or the inclination to read an erotic book, you probably do have time to listen to one. Most of us have some time in our day when we are plugged in, either to our i-pod or our laptop, and you might want to consider swapping a couple of play lists for an erotic novel or two.

Audio books are not for everyone, but if you have yet to give them a try, you might be pleasantly surprised by the results. I would strongly suggest starting with an erotic novel you may have already read, or perhaps an anthology that deals with a particular fantasy that you enjoy.

Erotic Fantasy Shopping Checklist

If this is your first time shopping for erotica, or you are unsure of how to pick your next book or DVD, there are a few things that you might want to consider before parting with your hard-earned cash.

Activities: What types of activities turn you on? Threesomes, couple-only sex, female masturbation, and lesbian scenarios are just a few examples that are available today. Having an idea of what activities or fantasies you enjoy can save you a lot of time when you are choosing erotica.

Orientation: Are you interested in any specific sexual orientation? (gay, straight, lesbian, transgender) or do you prefer a mix?

Point of View: Are you interested in a specific point of view, for example: a couple's perspective, a woman's perspective, or something else?

Genres: You can pull from mainstream movies here when making your choice. What type of movies/books interest you in general? Science fiction, mystery, and romance are just a few genres that are available in the erotic area today.

Language: Are you comfortable with sexually explicit language? Or do you prefer language to be a little less colorful?

Format: When it comes to erotic books, you can choose a novel, anthology, or a short story. When it comes to DVDs you may prefer a compilation of similar-themed scenes or a full-length feature film.

Quality: When it comes to erotic books it might be worth seeking out books that have won literary awards. With films, some are of a higher-quality production than others and you should ask yourself if this actually makes a difference to you.

Recommendations: Whilst you can't always ask your best friend for a recommendation when it comes to erotic choices, personal recommendations still hold a lot of weight. Failing that, though, there are plenty of good review websites for both written and visual erotica.

Electric Avenue: The Changing Face of Erotica/Porn

My first foray into porn was finding my father's stash of magazines in his closet, but things sure have changed since those days. With the advent of both the Internet and electronic readers, such as the Kindle, it's so much easier to find either porn or erotica in all its many and varied formats. The humble i-pod was how I first discovered audible erotica and I will admit to having spent many happy hours listening to some great erotica before showering and indulging in a good session of self-loving.

When it comes to erotic books, it's also much easier to read them in public without having to ever explain the cover or title of the book, thanks to e-readers.

Write it Up

So we've established that reading an erotic book can be a great way to get your mind in the mood, but have you ever considered writing it? You don't need to write your thoughts down as though you were going to seek an agent and publish them. It can be a fun exercise to simply scribble your innermost sexy thoughts into a diary, for example. Or you could try your hand at writing erotica – it can be a surprisingly sexy and liberating experience. If privacy is something that concerns you, try writing an erotic scene on your laptop and then simply delete it.

Do it Yourself

I've never met a smart phone that didn't have a camera in it. I'm not sure about you, but mine rarely leaves my side and I have been known to shoot an erotic video or two from the comfort of my bedroom. Oftentimes I will then just watch the video, practice some more self-loving before deleting the evidence, so to speak. Many women report that making a video of themselves masturbating has not only been a highly sexual experience but has also helped them see themselves in a whole new light. It's impossible to see what you look like when you orgasm, for the most part, but a video will help you appreciate the nuances of your own body. The advantage is you are the sole director of this movie, so you can choose whether you get close up and personal or take a more distant approach.

'I was alone, my roommate was away. I started to feel really horny while studying. Hmm… How would I do it this time? I sat there at my desk for a few minutes, touching my right breast with my cold fingers and coming up with a scenario. Oh, I needed it so bad! Then I went to the bathroom and washed my pussy, which was already wet from excitement. I took my mobile phone, set its camera to "record" and I hung it right next to the big mirror, so both the mirror and the phone were facing my bed.

Then I got completely naked. I sat on the bed, spread my legs and started to touch and massage my small white breasts, while watching myself in the mirror and also looking at the camera. Then I knelt on the bed. I squeezed my nipples and just watched my pink pussy in the mirror for a while and then I started touching it and rubbing my clit, while at the same time moving my hips in a circular motion. I put a finger in my cunt and squeezed my breast with my other hand, still moving my hips, and looking in the mirror. And boy, did that sight turn me on! Then I turned to the side so the camera was filming me from the right and I repeated all of those lovely things. After that I turned my ass to the camera and again rubbed my clit.

Then I squeezed my ass with my hands very hard.

Then I faced the camera again. I took my face-cleansing milk (which I had previously prepared, and washed the bottle so that it was cold) and just rubbed my cunt against the smooth plastic bottle, paying special attention to my lovely clit and touching my tits with quick motions with my free hand. I continued rubbing my clit with the face- cleanser bottle and massaging my tits, moving my hips in a circle, watching my reflection in the mirror. And then I came, mmmm… And what a great orgasm that was! After I came, I touched my pussy very gently for a while.

Then I got up and stopped the camera. Still naked, with a sensational feeling in my pussy, I lay on the bed and watched my own little dirty movie. Incredible feeling.'

Conclusion:

No matter how you choose to get yourself in the mood for some self-loving, it's always worth remembering that your mind is your most powerful sex organ. There is also no right or wrong way to get yourself in the right frame of mind for some self- loving, either. It's about taking what could otherwise be a normal situation and turning it into your own private sexy scenario.

CHAPTER 7

Basic Masturbation Techniques

I've said this before, but it is worth repeating once more, there is no right or wrong way to masturbate and the only way to figure out what works for your body is give yourself different techniques to try. At the end of the day, masturbation is inevitably about achieving an orgasm and many women report frustration when a particular technique or tool doesn't work for them. It's only by exploring your own body and being present in the moment that you will discover what does and does not work for you as an individual. So let's take a look at some of the more basic, or as I like to call them, easy-access, masturbation techniques that are available to you.

So what, exactly, is an easy-access masturbation technique, you might well ask? The answer is as simple as it sounds; one that requires no extra equipment other than your own body in order to cause you to experience an orgasm. I just realized I made that sound way more complicated than it actually needs to be, but I'm sure you get the gist. Basically, if it belongs to your body and it can help you masturbate, then you'll probably find it here.

Before we get there, though, let's talk about some basics as regards some simple things that you can do in order to get yourself in the right frame of mind for a masturbation session. Although we've already talked about fantasies and how powerful a sex aid our minds can be when it comes to masturbation, let's look at some practical ways to use that knowledge before we get into actual techniques.

Take Your Time

The thing about sex, even solo sex, is that many of us are in way too much of a hurry to just get rid of the itch we need to scratch. Of course, there are times when a quickie is simply all you need, but I would urge you to occasionally take some time out to simply explore other ways to masturbate. So often we are not present when we masturbate, as for so long it's been thought of as the second cousin to partnered sex, but the truth is by setting aside some time to explore your own body, what it likes and what it doesn't, the chances are that you can improve not only your solo sex life, but also your partnered sex life when, and if, you choose to have one.

Although I've been married for almost a quarter of a century, I am still a masturbator – and the reason is simple. Over the years my body has changed, my desires have changed, and so have those of my partner. By spending some time solo, I still discover things that turn me on, make me feel good, and these are things that I can then take back to my partnered-sex experiences.

So my suggestion is that a quickie is great when you just need that itch scratched, just as it would be if you were practicing partnered sex, but at least once in a while, slow down and take some time to enjoy your own body and all of the delights it has to offer. There are times when taking the time to care for ourselves and our own sexual needs can bring hidden pleasures to the forefront and, in turn, make us better mothers, partners, and just all-round people.

So, whether you are, like myself, an old hand at masturbation, or just starting out on the great sexuality journey, please take a moment to prepare yourself, both mentally and sometimes physically, to explore your own sexuality. Below are some ways in which you could prepare yourself for something more than a simple quickie:

'I have been single for a long time now, so have got masturbation on the brain. I can't go an hour without thinking about when I can get myself off. I really do enjoy masturbating and can go at myself for a good couple of hours at a time. If I have read these stories, then I become even worse and sometimes I will play with myself at least ten times. I love to get myself horny by taking my time and waiting until I can stand it no longer. So, by the time I actually start to finger-fuck myself, my clit is red-hot and throbbing to be poked. Like now, I am pressing my thighs so hard together that I think I will probably cum right away before I get a chance to insert anything in my pussy. Will have to leave this here now as my very juicy pussy is waiting for my fingers! And as I said, it is my normal routine to be masturbating furiously all night – starting right now.'

Date Night

Many of us have heard the advice given to couples who are looking to reconnect with one another. You know, where they are advised to set aside some time, get a babysitter, if required, and go on a date. When they return home, the idea is because they have taken the time to reconnect with each other outside of their normal environment. They will likely rediscover the connection that once bound them together.

The advantage of following the same advice if you are single should be pretty apparent, but in case it's not, let me enlighten you. Sometimes when we are single we become so focused on going out and finding the perfect mate, both sexually and from a lifelong standpoint, we forget that we will always live with ourselves, no matter how fulfilling a partnership may prove to be. Learning what we like as an individual, from both a sexual and emotional standpoint, can be a great place to start or restart the relationship we could be having with, well, ourselves.

For example, although I am very much committed to and in love with my partner, there are things that simply don't make him happy emotionally or sexually as they do me. The same is sometimes true in the bedroom, but we can generally work them out, as over the years we have learned to communicate very well. He does not enjoy going to art galleries and I do, for example. So, every now and then, I take a day out and go tour some galleries by myself, and a couple of nights a month I spend some time practicing some self-love. Just me, myself, and I. I look at this as an exercise in my own mental health, but it wasn't always like that. There were many years where I believed that taking time to work on myself, mentally and physically, was a selfish act. As I've grown older and, no, I won't say wiser, I've realized that those days are anything but selfish. They make me a better partner, lover, wife, and every other title that I, or society, choose to give ourselves or others.

When I get ready for a solo date night, I make sure I prepare for that evening just as I would if I was dating my partner. I spend time getting ready, I choose my wardrobe carefully, and I take time to focus on what pleases me. Sometimes I am in the mood for toys, sometimes porn, and sometimes I just get down and dirty, but whatever I decide to do that evening, I make sure that I have all the things in place before I begin my date. I have toys at the ready, my favorite porn movie queued up, or a couple of erotic books are placed strategically on my bedside table. By taking the time to prepare myself physically, I am getting in the mood emotionally as well. Being mentally prepared to give yourself the time that you deserve to explore the one thing that you ever truly

83

owned in life is as important as all the things that can be used to achieve an orgasm.

'I'm starting to get really wet, and it's all I can do not to put a finger to my clit and rub hard, but that will have to wait for now. Instead, I use my left hand to squeeze my breasts and feel the nipples through my thin shirt. I slip under the material and tease the small pink nipple until the right one is hard, then I do the same on the other side. I touch the tips of them with my fingertips and cup them for as long as I can take it, imagining I can feel someone licking circles and making them even harder.

My breathing gets shallower and I feel definitely wetter. I'm dripping and really anxious to feel some relief. I feel my clit throbbing and touch it with my index finger, press against it.'

Below you will find some of the most popular techniques that over the years Clitical visitors and myself have found worked for us when we do find time to spend some time with ourselves.

Touch Your Whole Self, Not Just Your Genitals

It's rare that when we have partnered sex we just get down and penetrative within the first 30 seconds of sex, even if we are looking for just a quickie. So many times, though, I hear the opposite is true when it comes to solo sex. Speaking for myself here, I require at least some foreplay before my sexual engines are really revved into high gear, and I'm sure this is true for many other women. Yet so many of us treat solo sex differently, as an experience where we simply concentrate all our energy and touches in the general area of our genitals.

I like to think of it this way; we are all an entire entity. Mind, body, and soul, as the saying goes, we are a collection of neurons, skin, bones, and nerve endings, and each one of those is in some way activated via the one simple action of touching them. Human touch is by far one of the most sexually charged tools we have in our sexual arsenal, but all too often it's forgotten.

How many times have you read or heard about a sex therapist offering advice to a couple that goes something along the lines of: For the next two weeks you can spend time simply touching each other's body. Lie next to each other naked and touch each other, but for the first week you are not allowed to touch your partner's genitals. The idea, of course, being that the said couple will get back in touch with each other, and after a week of simply touching, I'm willing to bet that for most couples the desire to touch their partner's genitals or have theirs touched by the end of the week has been at least stirred, if not completely resurrected.

Now let's go back to your solo sex practice and take this lesson and apply to those sessions for, say, a week. You can touch any part of your body but your boobs, vulva, backside, or vagina. You can use your fingertips to trace a pattern over your inner thighs, your neck, your calves – anywhere but the forbidden areas. I'm willing to bet by the end of the week you will have a burning desire to touch what was forbidden during this exercise, as well as a very heightened sense of just exactly how powerful your own touch can be.

'I love to take it nice and slow. Just regular old finger technique, but instead of following my urge to pump up and down really fast I go as slow as I can stand it. The anticipation builds and my climax is sometimes mind-blowing. I'm getting horny just thinking about it!'

Setting the Mood
On occasions, I like to take the time to spend some time making love to my own body, or, at the very least, reconnecting with it. Now this is not true every time I masturbate and there are times when I simply need to scratch an itch that either my mind, or someone

else, has created. During the times when I do like to prepare and set the mood, though, I often just do a few simple things that make my masturbation session a very pleasant experience.

Lights Out
I know I told you to turn the lights on in chapter two, but just forget I said that for a moment, and bear with me. Turning out the lights and then, perhaps, even setting a few candles around the room, can bring your masturbation experience to a whole new level. It allows you to concentrate on the movements you are making, the strokes that are turning you on, and your mind to wander off to those far-away places where pirates and princesses wander.

*Tip: I have a few small mason jars that are just right for holding tea lights or small candles. They offer a safer way to light up a room than simply burning candles in the buff. They work particularly well in the bathroom and add ambiance without any effort. *

One of our strongest senses, and one that is so often overlooked, is our sense of smell. If you have a partner, I'm sure you are familiar with the feelings that simply smelling the same cologne as they wear can evoke. There are plenty of other scents and aromas that can easily be used to set the mood for a session of self-loving, though. One of my favorite ways is to use scented candles or essential oils. The smell of coffee can transport me to a morning rendezvous with a lover, or remind me of the time I caught a glimpse of someone I once knew intimately whilst in the local coffee shop. Again, use the aroma to help conjure up a fantasy or a situation that makes you feel sexy.

Dress for the Occasion
Have you ever stopped to consider how long it takes you to get ready for a date, either with your current partner or a possible

new one? Now consider this: is it worth spending that time on yourself when you decide to participate in some self-love. I'm hoping that at least occasionally you will think that you are. I'm in no way suggesting that you need to get dressed up each and every time you decide to masturbate, but once in a while it can be a fun thing to do. It can also be a great aid when it comes to bringing a fantasy to life. On occasion I like to take this to a whole new level and dress up in a French maid's costume that I just happen to own, but that's another story entirely. Other times, I simply choose some lingerie that makes me feel good and dress in that. Like most things it's about the mood and setting the time aside to turn a simple self-love session into a special memory.

Turn It Up

Music can make for a great backdrop to help you get in the mood for some solo fun. I'm not sure about you, but sometimes I like a hard, heavy session and sometimes I prefer a softer gig. There is music to suit every mood and occasionally it can be fun to turn on your favorite album and sink into the music as you lie back and enjoy making your own sweet music.

Masturbation Techniques

So whilst you might think that solo sex is about just your genitals you might want to think again, which is why these basic masturbation techniques are not only centered around your clitoris and vulva. So let's start with your breasts and nipples as we embark on our exploration of the female form.

Breast Play

There are some women who report that they can come simply by manipulating their breasts and especially their nipples. I sadly am not amongst that group, but you might be! Stop shaking your head already, that is, unless you have already tried these techniques and they have had not produced an orgasm.

Even if nipple and breast play didn't make you come, the chances are the sensations made you feel good and sexy and at least got you in the mood, so to speak. Many women enjoy breast and nipple play as part of a solo sex session and so they should. There are several ways you can stimulate your breasts and that includes your nipples, as well as your vulva and clitoris. Many of the basic techniques and the way that you use your hands for self-stimulation, with the exception of a few, can be transferred to either vulva or breast for stimulation purposes. If you think of your nipples as the clitoris of your breasts, then you can hopefully see where the similarities between the two pieces of complex and wonderful anatomy exist. Yes, I know you can't feed a baby with your clitoris, but that aside, the similarities are still there!

'I start out by brushing my nipples over my shirt. Then I take my breasts out of my shirt and start rubbing my nipples harder and faster. When I can feel my pussy getting wet I start to pinch my nipples, which makes my pussy ejaculate. I keep doing this until I feel like I am going to explode unless I touch my clit. I stick my pointer finger slightly in my vagina and squeeze my clit between my thumb and middle finger, rubbing round and round until I come.'

Peg It
Many women enjoy breast stimulation by simply touching, pinching, or kneading them with their fingers or hands, whilst others find they need a little more pressure than their hands alone. You can buy nipple clamps that are built just for the purpose of providing such pressure, but there is a much simpler, not to mention cheaper, way to discover whether this type of stimulation works for you and your solo play. The humble clothes peg makes for a great nipple clamp! I prefer to use the wooden variety simply because this seems more organic than the plastic kind. I would caution you to start slowly here and not simply clamp the peg onto your nipple. If the pressure is too much, you can

loosen the spring on the wooden-type pegs by simply opening and closing the peg a few times, and then trying again until you get the correct pressure for pleasure.

'I am 46 years old and have been masturbating since age 13. I have always been very sexually active (including 3 marriages and several live-in relationships), yet masturbation has always been a large part of my life. I have a 27 year-old live-in now who was born way too late for his time and has actually taught me that solo-sex is wonderful, not a thing to be hidden. My favorite technique involves "lots" of KY, a dildo, a little "rush" for the head (something wacky to smoke beforehand will put you in an even "hornier" mood!), and the good ol' reliable fingers. My technique involves ass fucking for the big part. I like to lay on the bed and have a porn movie in for added effect…also have a mirror propped between my legs to see what I'm doing…this gets me even more excited. I begin by rubbing my clit and putting a finger in the vagina. I also like to use clamps on my nipples (they can stand a lot because of insensitivity after a breast reduction). I get myself worked up then lube up an 8 dildo with KY. This goes in the ass which is much more exciting to me than a vibrator in the vagina. During these episodes I am hitting off a bottle of Rush which really intensifies sex in any way. I fuck my ass hard with the left hand while rubbing horizontally across my clit with my right hand. I can hold off as long as I like and really have the most INTENSE orgasm ever! Because once I cum this way I am spent for at least an hour. (Just a little suggestion: prior to this an enema can be beneficial for "cleaner" results.) I think it's time I went to try out my "method".'

Touch Thyself
As we discussed before, touch is the greatest gift we have. We often give it to others, but prefer not to give it to ourselves. Again, I'm not talking about just touching your breasts or genitals, but your entire body. As we saw in chapter one (I'm really hoping

89

you've read that chapter by now!) all of our bodies are in some way erogenous zones that can help set the mood, before we even begin to touch the parts of our bodies that are generally thought of as sexual. If you did read chapter one, I hope that you will have tried out some of the exercises that I suggested there and if you did, then the chances are you know which parts of your body respond to your own touch the best.

Let Your Fingers Do the Walking

If you are as old as I am and from England, the chances are you remember this great tag line that was used by the marketing guys at the *Yellow Pages*. It is equally as true today as it was back then, and doubly so, when it comes to masturbation. The great thing about using your fingers and letting them do the walking is that they are directly connected to your brain and that should make them your number-one tool in your masturbation arsenal. After all, they are always, well, handy, whether you are in the mood for a slower session or simply a quickie.

'I'm staying on my parent's couch until I move in a few weeks, so I have to wait until everyone is asleep and the house is quiet. I just reached down and began stimulating my clit. Varying the intensity and speed of rubbing, I came in about ten minutes and then settled down to go to sleep.'

Under Pressure

Touch is not just about where you choose to touch yourself, but rather often the pressure that you apply when you do so. A light, playful touch will produce different sensations to one where you grab, roll, or pinch your breasts or clitoris, after all.

'I prefer to lie with buttocks on the edge of the bed, with legs hanging off the edge of the bed, back flat on the bed. I pull the lips back and use my index finger to massage the inner portion of my clit. As I

get more excited, I pull more tautly on the outer lips and increase the speed and pressure.'

Circles of Desire

I enjoy a circular motion on both my breasts and my vulva when I am using my fingers for solo play. For my breasts, I generally start with a wider circle and then begin to narrow it down as my desire for more touch begins to grow. It's also fun to start with smaller circular motions and then work outward into ever-bigger circles. You could also try spiraling motions around your breasts and nipples and see how your body reacts to each type of touch. I also like to increase and decrease the pressure I apply to my skin at various times.

You can do the same thing with your inner thighs as I detailed above and as you get closer to your vulva, decrease the circles and lighten up your touch in anticipation of circling your clit. I like to circle around my clitoral hood a little, until my good friend is exposed and then, if the mood takes me, touch my actual clitoris and see what happens. The other thing I would recommend here is that you might want to apply some lubricant to your vulva at some point and, again, this can make for some very different, but often satisfying, sensations.

'I just read your article about masturbating. I have a method I would like to share that works for me. I lie flat on my back with both of my legs spread widely apart. Sometimes I have one leg up and the other lying flat on the bed or bent a little to the side. Using my pointer and middle finger, I slowly go down to my pussy and circle the hole to lubricate the two fingers. Then, I move up to my clit and put the two fingers either just above the clit or beside it, just barely touching it. Like, I am on it but not on top of it, so the intensity is not too intense. Then, I move my fingers in a circular motion, starting off slow and then moving faster as I feel myself getting ready to come – like

the peeing sensation. I also play with my tits and nipples to add to the excitement. Many times, I also think about someone eating my pussy out and picture them in between my lips lapping away. I read visualizing someone inside of you or eating can make an instant orgasm. It works for me. That's all I am adding right now.'

Stroke It

A simple stroke seems like the obvious thing to do when you masturbate, but I want you to think in terms of type of stroke here as opposed to simply petting the cat. Think about it for a second. There are all types of different strokes in the world and by varying your choices you can add to or decrease the pleasure to each of your solo sessions. There are long strokes, there are short strokes, there are the kinds of strokes you use when applying eye liner, you know the intermittent strokes, where you do a quick dash followed by another and yet another. There are vertical and horizontal strokes and there are, as we discussed before, circular strokes. By trying different types of strokes and also the pressure with which you apply them, you may just open up a whole new world of sensations. In fact, I'm willing to bet that you will do just that.

Then, of course, the next thing we should consider is exactly where we place those strokes and the different sensations they can cause. Many women have found that one side of their clitoris or labia may be more sensitive than the other and this is a perfect way to experiment and find out of this is true for you. Try stoking just one side first and seeing how your body reacts and then simply switching sides. I'm pretty sure that one will produce more pleasure than the other, but the only way to find out for yourself is to try. Of course, you can place your fingers on both sides of your clitoris and simply enjoy the sensations.

'In bed on my back I gently start rubbing my pubic area, then slowly

begin, with one finger, rubbing the side of my vagina. Once I'm excited enough, I stroke my vagina and concentrate on the upper half (clit area). I then enjoy rubbing my clit in a circular motion until orgasm. Occasionally I have penetrated my vagina with my fingers, but I do not require the penetration for orgasm.'

Tap It

Many women report that tapping their vulva, nipples, or anus can be a very pleasurable experience. Personally, this is not something I enjoy, with the exception of my nipples, but, that said, it wasn't until I tried it I knew I didn't enjoy it, so please don't let it stop your experimenting.

'Lie down flat on your back. Lick the fingers and thumbs of both hands and use them to massage your breasts, kneading them while pinching and pulling your nipples. Do this until your nipples are hard, then move one hand down your torso and spread your legs apart. Use that hand to gently massage your clit until you feel like you're going to orgasm. When you feel this way, move your other hand to your slit and insert two fingers into your vagina. Find your g-spot and move your fingers, tapping it repeatedly while increasing the pressure and speed used on your clit. When you feel like you're about to burst, begin massaging your clit with three fingers, rubbing them against it and pressing hard. Do this until you orgasm.'

Rub It

Rubbing your vulva, clitoris, boobs, or nipples, will not produce a genie, you have my word on that, but it might produce some great sensation, and if you're really lucky an orgasm may ensue. Just as with all the other forms of finger-touching, applying various pressures to the rubbing action can produce different sensations, as you would expect. You can also vary the speed at which you rub for even more sensation.

'I tend to lie on my back, relax, and start to slowly finger my vagina with my legs bent and wide apart. When I have a bit of cum on my fingers I rub my clit slowly, then when I get used to the feeling I rub it vigorously – trust me, it will make you moan with pleasure! But I find it even more orgasmic and longer-lasting if you rub your clit dry. It is just WOW!'

Pinch and Roll

Pinching and rolling either your nipples or clitoris can be a great combination of moves. Start with placing your forefinger and thumb over your clit or nipple and gently pinch it, then roll off to one side or the other. If you find that it is not enough pressure, apply more pressure until you find the combination that works for you.

'I'm sitting here reading all of these techniques and I can feel my clit swelling up in my panties. It's all tingly and wet down there and I can't wait to go and rub my pussy when I'm finished here. For me, the anticipation is one of the best parts! My favorite technique has always been pinching. I lie down on my bed on my back, and spread my butt cheeks open to leave my twat fully exposed. Then I run my fingers around the outer part of it, and over my nipples. If you barely touch them, it feels amazing. Eventually, I start pinching my nipples and then sliding my fingers all around my clit. It gets very slippery down there so I always only apply a light touch. As I get a little bit hornier I'll start pinching my clit with my thumb and index finger… faster then slower, firmer then softer. When I come, my nipples harden up and my pussy gets unimaginably wet. Sometimes I watch what I'm doing with a mirror. Every now and then, I'll fuck myself afterwards with my favorite dildo.'

Dual Stimulation

All of the above types of movements can be used to great effect in unison on your nipples and vulva, clitoris and breasts, or any

94

combination you like at the same time. I like to think of all these types of movements as the standard fare at the buffet. There is a movement or combination of movements that will suit everyone. After all, you have not one hand but two and being able to use them both can be a real bonus and it's sort of a shame to waste them, when you think about it.

Water Techniques
H2O or, as it's more commonly known, water, can be put to great effect when it comes to self-pleasure. After all, we all shower or bath pretty much every day and often the bathroom is the one place in the house where we all have locks. Showers are good for hiding the sounds that can be associated with a hot and steamy self-love session as well, which is always a bonus, in my book. If you're lucky enough to have access to a spa or hot tub, again you can put water to good use for your own unselfish sexual pleasure. Of all the things I look for in a property, whether I'm considering renting or buying, is a great bathroom, and preferably one with a decent shower. Many showers come with detachable shower heads and if you are lucky enough to have one of these you can find you may use it for things other than simply getting clean. If you do not have access to a detachable shower head, fear not, a simple faucet can also provide many hours of sexy fun as you will see as we begin to explore some of the more popular water techniques that I and many Clitical visitors have tried over the years.

Shower Me With Kisses
A shower head is useful in many ways, but one of its most common uses amongst women is to provide pleasure. I like the detachable kind that can be used separately from the faucet on account of its long, flexible hose. This offers many more self-pleasure possibilities but a fixed-head type of shower can also be utilized in the pursuit of some good clean fun.

Have you ever stood under the shower when you have been aroused and noticed that as the water trickles down over your body, you start to tingle, your sense of touch replicating your arousal? Water can be an amazing tool when it comes to self-love and harnessing it is incredibly simple.

You are likely already naked when you step into the shower stall. If your intention is to play with the water, then simply play. This is where you can take real advantage of a detachable shower head if you have one. Spend time guiding the water over your naked body, find a water temperature that works for you and spend some time exploring your own body. No one is watching or judging you, it's time to open up your mind and your body and unlock the sensations it can provide.

As you become more aroused, allowing the water to travel over your body, move the head around and slowly bring it down so that is angled between your legs. It might be easier to place one leg on the edge of the tub, if possible, at this point. Now I want you to begin exploring your vulva with the water. You will discover that by varying the distance between your vulva and the shower head you can produce various sensations, some more pleasurable than others. There are no rights or wrongs here, just what works for you, remember.

If your shower head has a massaging head function you can have some fun playing with the various pulsations it can produce, Some of these you may find too intense if you are new to shower-head play and I would recommend you use them sparingly first. Try directing the water to your inner thighs, for example, before you allow it to travel to your vulva. Bear in mind you will have a free hand here and can use this to tease your nipples, or stoke the rest of your body here. Remember that, as always, there are no rights or wrongs here, just simply what feels good.

'I had some more fun in the shower the other day. My pussy was aching for some attention, so when I stepped into the shower I slipped two fingers past my pussy lips and teased my clit, mmm so wet. After that, I stopped for the time being and washed my hair, and then lathered my entire body with soap, and giving my breasts and pussy special attention when I lathered them. I brushed over my breasts with my fingers and then pinched them, getting them nice and hard. And then I slid my hand down to my pussy again, smearing my soap and juices all over me. The hot water teased me so much when I rinsed off, making my nipples extra perky and sensitive.

When I couldn't take it any longer, I sat down on the edge of the tub. I used the shower head to tease my nipples again, watching them harden and squeezing them, feeling myself throb with anticipation. Then I move the head down to my pussy, moving water in circles around the outside first. Then I spread my legs to expose my wet, aching pussy and let the water run over my clit, oh it felt soo good ... I found the spot that made my pussy clench in want, and let the water tease me there. I started to buck from pleasure, and then turned the jets on high, sending me into a frenzy.

I could imagine two of you girls licking in between my thighs, your tongues clashing, flicking, and sucking all over me, gets me so hot ... Telling me how I'm such a dirty girl and that you want me to cum for you, giving you all my juices, pinching and rolling my nipples in your fingers while you lick and suck on my aching pussy. Suddenly I'm cumming and my pussy is sending shock waves all throughout my body, making me moan and thrust for you. I love how intense cumming in the shower is!'

Spa With Me

If you are lucky enough to own, or have access to, a hot tub, you are likely familiar with the power of water jets already. Many Clitical visitors have reported that for them this was how they first discovered masturbation and how good it can feel. The technique itself is a simple one and can, in fact, be employed whether you are alone or with company, but if it's your first time trying I would strongly urge you to make sure you are solo unless you are messing with a trusted partner.

For this technique you simply place your vulva over the water jets of the hot tub. Yes, it's as simple as it sounds. The only difficult thing here is that different tubs have different power ratios when it comes to their jets. Some of the cheaper plug-and-play- type spas are not quite as powerful as their more expensive counter- parts, but don't let that stop you enjoying the sensations they are both more than capable of producing. I would strongly suggest keeping your underwear or swimming costume on as you explore the powerful jets, as they can act as a useful barrier to what can sometimes be sensations that are a little overwhelming at first. You also have a choice here, you can back up to the jets and allow the water jet to glide between your legs and hit your vulva and clitoris in the process, or you can spread your legs and allow a full-on water assault to occur. The first option is obviously a little more subtle and I would recommend it for first-time water play, to be honest, as the second option can provide too much stimulation if you are not used to it. Start slowly and, as always, find what works for you and your body.

'After I visit Clitical.Com and my pussy is wet and ready to go, I walk outside to our hot tub naked. My secret desire is to have a neighbor watch me in the hot tub as I spread my lips and let the hot tub jet hit my clit. Just as I am about to come and my clit is huge, I move away from the jet and finger myself or let the jet shoot up my ass. Anal is one of my favorite positions with my husband. The pressure feels so good. I think about all of the women on here flicking their clits and using their vibrators to get themselves off and think about having one of them touch my pussy until I come all over (maybe someday I will be with another woman). I put my clit as close to the jet as I can and let the orgasm build again. Sometimes I can

stay outside and come over and over. After this I go back to being a
working mom and wife.'

Faucet Fun

So you don't have a shower? Not a problem. You can use your humble bath faucet for your own pleasure and it requires no extra tools or fancy equipment to do so. If you opt for this technique, you need to check your water temperature. I like it tepid or on the cooler side than many Clitical readers have reported, but determine a water temperature that works for you. Now you just scooch down into the tub, so you are lying on your back with your legs spread and raised up toward the faucet. Whilst this might sound, and even feel, a little awkward the first time, it's really not that hard. You have to just find a position that works for you and one where the water will stream over your vulva. Some women report that they like to use their hips to push upward, which in turn enables them easier access to the water and to better position themselves so the stream is running directly across their clitoris. Others prefer a more subtle approach, but, as with everything masturbation-wise, there is no right or wrong way, just the way that works for you.

'I just had to share somewhere about my amazing orgasmic experi-
ences. I am new to the masturbation world, but I have found that it
does wonders for me when I'm very stressed or just sexually aroused.
I usually can only get excited in the shower or the tub but that's
okay because it is more private anyway. I like to lie under the faucet
with the water pouring onto my clit while rubbing fiercely with two
fingers. I never knew how amazing this would be and this site, along
with others, really helped me to find how to please myself in such
an amazing way!'

Rub-a-Dub Tub

You can put the bathtub to good use without the need for water by simply using its edge to slide along. I would recommend using a good lubricant during this process as it tends to make the experience a little more comfortable. Just swing one leg over the edge of the tub, so you are straddling the edge, and move up and down along the edge so your vulva is rubbing the edge of the tub. By varying the length of your strokes it's possible to produce a great many different sensations with this technique. It also leaves your hands free so you can touch other parts of your body and that always makes for an interesting experience.

'Sit on the edge of the tub with your legs on either side. Rock back and forth and grind your pussy. I usually go wild with this one. Another technique I use is when I have to pee badly, I hold it and then masturbate. The feeling is sooooo intense.'

Laundry Lover

If you own a washing machine at home this is a fun technique that has the potential to make washday a lot more fun. By positioning your vulva on the edge/corner of the washing machine and turning it to a spin cycle, it is possible to achieve stimulation. Personally, I've found older machines can be more efficient when it comes to masturbating.

Look No Hands Techniques

There are several techniques that require either your feet, heels, or some other part of your body as opposed to the usual 'use your hands' techniques. The great advantage these techniques have is that they can often be deployed in normal situations. You could, for example, be sitting at your office desk or at lunch and deploy any of the following below without the risk of being detected, unless of course you are a screamer like me, and orgasm is now accompanied by a banshee-like moan that would probably wake the dead. In some ways these techniques could be considered 'stealth' methods, but they can also be used and practiced when you are alone.

Come To Heel

This technique is as much about position as it is actual masturbation and, as the name suggests, it involves your heel. All you need to see if this works for you is to simply sit with one leg tucked beneath you. Now you rock from side to side and allow your heel to do the work for you as it rubs against your clitoris and vulva. Some women can come quite easily whilst doing this, but it can be a little tricky for others. As with all the techniques here, though, it costs nothing to experiment and to see if this will work for you. If you discover you can't come this way, you can try adding in a thin jeans seam and see if that has more effect on you.

'I found a while ago the heel of your foot in the right place is just perfect. To use my laptop, the only place I can sit is cross-legged on my bed and I soon found my heel sitting in this position was in the perfect place to rub me and all I do is move my foot a bit and it has the added advantage that if someone comes in I look as if I am only sitting cross-legged, so no odd comments. I find it does not do too much, but at least starts things off nicely.'

Squeeze Me, Please Me

This is another technique that can be practiced whilst you are sitting in your chair and, again, some women report coming long and hard from this one. All you do is sit in your chair, as you normally would, then you squeeze your buttocks and, in turn, your pelvic muscles until you find a rhythm that works for you. This technique turns me on, but I will admit to never having orgasmed from it, but that's fine because for me, as it should be for you, it's about the journey not the destination and not every technique will work for you.

'I am on my way home. A grey landscape hurtles by as the train speeds down the track. My seat rattles, going from a gentle throb to a banging clatter. From absent daydreaming, I move to consciousness.

To this rough movement. To the throttle of the engine that feels like a giant vibrator. I move ever so slightly in my seat. Between my legs, my flower unfurls. I close my eyes and feel the warmth rise. My clit awakens. I clench my muscles as the vibration shoots through me like an electric shot. Oh my God! This makes the feeling grow. It mounts. Becomes intense. I cross my legs. Tightly. So tightly that the pressure builds on my clit. It fights back, pressing up against my thighs. Threatening to explode. But no, it can't. No, I can't. I mustn't come in public. My vulva is on fire. The heat rises from my belly, flushing my face, making my breath come shallow and fast. I spread my legs just slightly. Just enough to free the inner petals of my beautiful cunt. Through my knickers, through my jeans, they graze the seat. I press down to meet the vibration head-on. A moan slips my lips. I catch myself. But nothing can stop the hot fluid that is pouring out. I can feel it. Unable to contain myself, I lean forward, splaying out my buttocks, pressing my vulva into the seat. Pressing my asshole into the seat. My perineum into the seat. Sweet agony. This train ride is two hours long. How can I last? My clit feels hard, rock-like. Although I cannot touch myself, I can feel that I am drenched, as are my pants. A deep ache takes shape inside my empty cunt. It reminds me that I need to be filled, to be pummelled, to be stretched. I clench and unclench my muscles, feeling the burning build at the entrance to my vagina. I am flushed and hot. My breasts feel imprisoned in their bra. My ovaries begin to ache with longing. So, too, the muscles of my groin. Deep inside my cunt, my cervix feels engorged, as if begging to be touched. This pleasure is unbearable. Larger than me. Stronger than me. Right now, all of me is my cunt. Just my cunt. My beautiful, burning cunt.

At last, I reach my station. I lope down the street, racing home. Once inside, I slam the door shut and run upstairs to my bedroom, tearing my clothes off as I go. Naked, I throw myself onto the duvet covering the bed. It feels cool against my skin. I sink my face into it. My nipples harden. My belly sinks into the softness beneath me. My legs writhe and spread. At last, I can moan. Out loud. In desperation,

I clutch at the duvet, scrunching it up, shoving it madly between my legs. Something, anything to quieten this feeling. I grind into it, grunting animal-like as I do so, my vulva and my ass humping its coolness. I jerk my ass a thousand times, like a madwoman. Like a woman on fire. My clit is all that matters now. Yes, in and out, in and out. Yes, yes, yes. Oh God, yes. My clit feels sore, but I love it. I love it. I love it. My clit is my being. It is alive. It is strong. It is powerful. About to burst. And then I cannot hold back any longer. My entire cunt explodes into the duvet. The orgasm shoots through me from foot to head, making me gasp for air. Paroxysms of pleasure. I shriek as the lava gushes out of me. Shaking me. Making my feet curl. Like a waterfall, the tension drains at last. Exhausted, I lie quiet for a moment or two. Then I notice that the duvet is drenched. Have I peed or have I squirted? I do not know. It does not matter. I raise the wet duvet to my lips. It tastes of salt. Of my clit. Of my cunt.'

Conclusion:
I think the techniques above are pretty much self-explanatory and, as you can see, the variations are infinite. You can choose to combine any one with another and in the process discover which of them work best for you.

CHAPTER 8

Anytime, Anywhere!

It's easy to think of masturbation as simply a means to an end, with that end resulting in an orgasm. With a little thought it can be so much more than that, though. Just as you can, and should, learn to explore your body through self-pleasure you can easily do the same simply by changing your surroundings or the position in which you choose to masturbate. In this chapter we will be taking a closer look at how and where those changes can be made.

Positions Please
A quick flick through any glossy magazine and you are likely to find at least one article talking about sex and, more importantly, sexual positions. Doggy style, cowboy, and missionary are by far the most common partnered sexual positions. The basic principle being: by changing your positions or that of your partner you can change the feeling that you both achieve.

Yet people rarely apply the same logic to solo sex and I have yet to figure out why. I'm here to tell you the biggest discovery I found when I discovered self-loving was that by simply changing the position of my body I could change the feelings and, in some cases, the type of orgasms I could achieve.

Lie Back and Relax
This is probably the most familiar of all the masturbation positions. It's the way many of us start to masturbate, by just lying back on the bed or sofa, or even in the tub, and beginning to explore all the delights that self-pleasure has to offer. The advantages of this position are that it is easy to achieve access to most parts of the body and requires little effort, leaving us free to enjoy the sensations we choose to create with our fingers, toys, or whatever else we decide to use.

'First I read a very erotic book or magazine while in the bathtub, then I let the water flow at a very slow rate and lie on my back (the water level is fairly low) and place my genital area under the water flow. I use one hand, usually the left, to "open" the area then lie back and fantasize! The results are great! Sometimes I use the ribbed end of my hairbrush if I feel like I need a little more, or if I am really frustrated. Also a hand-held shower head with a real fast pulsating stream works great!'

Kneel and Heel
This is one of my personal favorite positions when I'm indulging in some self-love. I simply kneel on the bed or on the floor and play as usual. This can be the perfect position for dildo play especially with the type of dildo that has a flared base that allows it to stand flat on a surface. Simply place the dildo on a stable surface, kneel over it, and take your pleasure. Adding a dildo with a suction-cup base can take kneeling to a whole new dimension, by the way. I love the fact that kneeling allows me to play with my hands free, allowing me full access to any other parts of my body. I sometimes like to use a clitoral massager whilst I have an object such as a dildo inserted. The reason I mention the heel here

is that for some women kneeling and sitting backward onto their heel, and then rocking back and forth, can produce a satisfying orgasm and is something you might want to try.

'I find that using the heel of my foot to get off on brings me a mind-blowing orgasm... Lie across the bed face down. Pull up one knee, tucking it between your breasts. Position yourself so your clit rests on the heel of your foot. Movements – up/down, circular, fast, slow – while maintaining contact with your heel bring an intense O. A little lubricant or toothpaste on your heel intensifies the sensation.... Flexibility is a plus...Time to take my shoes off...'

Stand to Attention
As the name suggests, standing-up masturbation, which can, I will admit, prove to be a little tricky, can again create a very different sensation within your body, especially as you peek over the crest of an orgasm. If space is restricted, for some reason, or you are playing in a shower stall, for example, the standing-up position is one that you might want to give a shot.

'Since I was 15 I always masturbated in bed or in the bathtub (I'm 22 today). But recently I sort of got bored with this and began trying different positions. I found that cumming while standing up is incredible! I'd recommend anyone to try this. The only problem is that it's kind of hard to reach my clit when I'm standing, so I usually start out as usual, lying down. I get myself really aroused, until I'm approaching the edge. Then I pause, sit up, and swing my legs off the bed onto the floor. I start diddling again until I'm very ready to cum. When I'm that close, I get to my feet and have the orgasm standing. It's great and it gives a really weak-in-the-knees and lightheaded feeling. Sometimes I can still feel the effect hours later.'

Doggy Style
This position is basically where you position yourself on all-fours

and works well if you have a dildo with a suction cup and a tiled bathroom wall, in my experience. You can simply stick the dildo to the bathroom wall and back up to it. You can also do this if you have a bed or a sofa that falls at the right height. You can simply slip your tool of choice between the covers, back up on all-fours and enjoy to your heart's content. Of all the positions, I feel this one is the most difficult to achieve, but in my opinion it's well worth the effort.

1) First take a shower.

2) Jump in bed.

3) Think of something erotic, like my boyfriend's hard dick, to get myself wet.

4) Start touching my pussy and spread the lube.

5) Get into my favorite position, the doggy.

6) Imagine that my boyfriend is behind me and I'm showing off my pussy to him.

7) I run my finger up and down the slit of my pussy and pretend it's my boyfriend's dick.

8) When tension starts to build, I insert a finger into my pussy and rub my clit with my thumb. Then bang, I cum in waves.'

Squat for Fun
This position involves squatting, as the name suggests, and can be a great addition to your position arsenal and is one that is often overlooked. You can choose to either practice a full-out squat or as the lady who so eloquently describes her own technique below

does. This position is basically a variation of the doggy style, but can make for some interesting orgasms, for sure.

'Ever since I can remember, I've used pretty much the same position while pleasuring myself. When I was a teenager I used to think I was odd — that it was a strange position, that I was probably freaky, and that the vast majority of women do it lying on their backs, or something. (Now I'm sure I'm not alone; I saw a lover once assume an unlikely position while he masturbated, with his legs way up in the air.) I sort of sit on my ankles and hunch over, lifting myself up a bit. There's something satisfying about the balance of body weight. Anyway, once sitting there, with my right hand cupped a little, I bunch together my fingertips to make little circles just above my clitoris, on the hood – the glans is too sensitive. With my other hand (also cupped a little with the fingertips bunched together) I press my fingertips against the opening to my vagina, but with the labia closed over that part so it's like hard pressure instead of penetration. The combination is great, because with my left hand I can feel every contraction as I orgasm, and somehow my hand feeling the contractions lets my brain sense them in my vagina more clearly. I'm really "there" with each contraction in a way I can't quite always be with a penis inside instead. They're like waves rippling throughout me.'

Belly Up, Or in This Case, Down

Lying on your belly is a lot more popular than you might think as a masturbation position. I will admit it's not a position that I've ever been comfortable in, but according to the poll I conducted on Clitical, it's a lot more popular than I thought it would be. This is a simple position, which requires you to, well, lie on your belly with your hand between your thighs and do what you do best: touch yourself in whichever way feels good for you.

'Depends on the tool in use! With a toy, I prefer on my back relaxing, with my fingers I prefer in my car as I'm driving, if I'm masturbatory without touching my vagina I prefer prostrate on my belly.'

Places and Spaces

It's so easy to limit ourselves when it comes to sex to, well, the bedroom and, more specifically, the bed. Of course, it's true that the bed is a great place and the bedroom a great space to partake in some self-loving, but by thinking outside the box or, in this case, the bed, the possibilities can be limited only by your imagination.

By changing your surroundings or looking at them in a different light, you can often add some much-needed umpph to your self-love routines. Think of it this way, if you were with a partner for a long time, you might get bored if you limited yourself to sex in the bed or bedroom. Partners may come and go, but one thing is for sure, you are going to have to live with your body, well, as long as you live, and hopefully that will prove to be a long time! So why not pay attention to the places and spaces you make love to yourself in, just as you would in any long-term relationship, because, after all, this is the longest relationship you will ever be in.

It's not hard to change your perspective on things. For example, I just took a walk around my house and I suggest you do the same after you've read this chapter. While I was touring my own home I was looking at all the possibilities and I will detail some of them here.

It's my bathroom and I'll clean it as fast as I want to: If, like me, you have kids, the bathroom is likely the only place in the house where you have true privacy. Lock the door and go to town tonight. Even moms deserve some self-loving time and the great thing about the bathroom is not only does it have a lock, it probably has a shower, tub, and toilet. You can use any of these three objects to help you enjoy your alone time. Let me explain further:

The bathtub, should be pretty self-explanatory, but you can do so much more than simply lie in a tub full of water. You can use the edge of the tub, for example, to slide across for a different sensation. Add in some waterproof lubricant and see what sensations you can create. If you choose to lie in the tub you have more possibilities. For example, place your feet above the faucet and let the water trickle or gush from the faucet onto your legs and your vulva. For many women this is a great way to orgasm.

You could simply add a waterproof toy into the mix here and get down and not so dirty. It's worth noting here that there is a difference between a waterproof toy and a splashproof one. I suggest you check that your toy is waterproof before you use it in the bathroom – just for safety's sake. Also do NOT use toys that connect to a power outlet in the bathtub.

Another popular way to get off in the bathtub requires a clean, empty water bottle, the kind that you squeeze. You can pick these up in your local Walmart for less than a buck. Simply fill them with water and squeeze onto your vulva. The sensations can be quite exquisite and, with a little practice, result in an orgasm.

You've probably heard that a detachable shower head is a girl's best friend and it's true. Not only are they great if you need to wash your hair without taking a full shower, they are great for getting off with. Spend some time getting to know your best friend, use it to tease and please all of your body, finishing by applying it to your clitoris. I personally have a power-head attachment and have been known to use it on many occasions.

Now take a look at your bathroom sink. See that electric toothbrush? That could be your new best friend, as many women have found out. According to many of Clitical's visitors they make for great vibrators, so much so I have thought about purchasing shares in Oral B. I do strongly suggest that you buy one for your teeth and another for your clitoris, though. Another handy found toy can be a vibrating razor. Take off the head and voila! I'm sure you are getting the idea, by now, that opportunities for self-love abound everywhere, so take another look around your bathroom and see what ideas you can come up with.

You can choose to partake of a quickie in the bathroom or you can set the scene. Once in a while I will pull out all the stops and bring out the scented candles, my very best fluffy towels, and spend some serious time with, well, myself.

'Since I have no toys, I now use a Venus razor handle and a Hummingbird electric flosser. First, you find that "sweet spot" near your clit, and when you find it, keep the vibrator on there. Then, insert the handle of the razor into you. While keeping the vibrator on, begin the move the handle in and out of yourself, slow at first, and then get faster and faster as you go. You cum soon enough, and keep it up and you may orgasm.'

It's Getting Hot In Here: I'm sure you can already envision lots of possibilities for self-loving as you look around your kitchen, but have you thought about looking in the fridge and seeing what takes your fancy in there? Zucchinis, carrots, European cucumbers are a few veggies that come to mind that can provide a lot of fun. My first- ever dildo was actually a zucchini that I pared down to resemble the shape of a penis. I added a condom and voila! There you go – one home-made fun toy.

There are plenty of other found toys that can be used in the kitchen. I've heard of women improvising with rolling pins and handles from various kitchen utensils. The one thing I will say

111

here: please use your common sense. Bottles may look like fun, but a trip to the ER is not – and it does happen.

I love the textures and various surfaces that are found in the kitchen and many are worth exploring. Lying on a cold tile floors can create a different sensation to that of lying on your cool bed. Equally, the wooden/tiled surface of a kitchen table can offer a different sensation.

The freezer is another place that is worth some exploration whilst in the kitchen. Sensation play is not limited to being between partners. There is no reason why you can't use the ice in that freezer to tease yourself, or if you have no ice a bag of frozen peas, while not sexy, will suffice and do the job just as well.

My Vivacious Living Room: Now we are here, take a look around. See that sofa? That is an ideal place to lie back, relax, and let your fingers do the walking. Equally the comfy chair that your partner loves can offer a great place to, well, spread your legs and simply enjoy. The coffee table or floor also offers a chance to get in some self-love. Now doesn't that sound so much more fun than watching the TV?

That pillow over there... Yep, the one that cost you an arm and a leg and you've never liked it since. Well you can put that to good use and spend a little time humping it and showing it who really is the boss here.

Some women have found a new use for their remote controls and turned them into found sex toys. I've personally not tested this one out because, well, I think it would be extremely difficult to clean the remote after some playtime. If it floats your boat, though, why not give it a try yourself?

112

'It was the first warm day of spring and I got lunch with my friends and had a few drinks. I came back to my apartment to get ready to go out that night, and found my roommate gone. I went to the kitchen for water, and for some reason (probably the margaritas) I slipped down the top of my strapless dress and then my bra and let my tits out. They're so big and round and I love playing with them. And all of a sudden, I was so horny that I knew I needed to masturbate.

I literally dropped my panties right there in the kitchen and started fingering myself. I'd never needed to touch my pussy so badly; I was so wet that my fingers were slipping on my hard clit. I leaned against the pantry and started rubbing myself, but it was a little hard to maneuver standing up.

I have a big armchair in the living room, so I sat down in that. I usually have to masturbate quietly in my own room so my roommate doesn't notice, but since she was at work, I was free. I kept my dress on but let my tits stay free so I could play with them while I stroked my clit. I let myself be as loud as I wanted, moaning at every touch.

I knew I needed a little more, though, so I slipped two fingers inside myself and started rubbing my g-spot. One hand on my rock-hard nipples, one hand in my dripping-wet pussy, I was masturbating myself to bliss. I didn't even know that I could be as loud as I was, practically screaming as I finger-fucked myself.

Then, all of a sudden, I squirted. Even though squirting porn is my favorite, I'd only managed to do it once before. And now, my pussy was literally gushing, filling my hand and dripping down onto my dress and the hardwood floor. Just feeling that sweet pussy juice all over me made me cum harder than I have in a long time. My whole body arched up off the chair and I was screaming and moaning and cursing at the top of my lungs. My pussy was pulsing for a good 30 or 45 seconds by the time I finally calmed down. I lay there for a few minutes, just feeling how wet every part of me was.

And the kicker? I realized my apartment window was open, meaning everyone heard my moaning. And the guys next to me can see into my living room, and I caught a glimpse of one of them watching me as I came down from my orgasm. Wonderful.'

Dining-Room Divas

There are quite a few things that you can have some fun with in this room as well. Why not lie on your dining-room table and pleasure yourself, or sit on the formal chair and be not quite so formal.

Oftentimes there are candles found in the dining room and they can make for some sexy fun, as long as you use some common sense. Most candles are straight and are therefore not suitable for anal play. As far as vaginal play is concerned, they can be inserted, but as with all found toys, please remember that cleanliness is next to godliness here and use some common sense.

'Honestly, I have to confess this. So I've been a bit naughty…Okay super naughty! My girlfriend refuses to play with me any more until I let her move me into her new apartment. So I've been sexually frustrated and decided to look up some fun things to do lol. So first thing I did was get completely naked and sat in front of my tinted dining-room window (you know, the kind that you can see out but they can't see in?) on my dining table and lathered myself in my favorite rose oils, getting myself aroused as I watched many people taking walks down my street and the neighbors across the street having a garage party. I rubbed the oil on my pussy, then took a wonder cream to my clit, getting it nice and swollen from being so horny as it peeked from my pussy lips. I took a paddle that was lying with the other toys I had and spread my legs wide in front of the window. I pinched a nipple hard, stretching it out as I smacked my inner thighs and pinched the other nipple. I stopped and took one dildo into my tight, sopping pussy and took a piece of ice and shoved it deep in my ass, I began to smack my aching clit with the paddle, only lightly at first, but before I could really get into it and try out more kinky things the kitchen door opened and…'

114

Love Me, Love my Bedroom: So now we are back where we started. Take another look around and see if you see this room in a different light now we have taken our house tour. Hopefully you can see more than the bed as a possibility now. If those pillows looking seriously inviting, no problem, why not try humping them instead of lying back on them? For many women who have cuddly toys in their bedroom, this can offer their first foray into self-pleasure. You may be able to put that favorite teddy to a whole new use. It just takes a little imagination.

'When I am alone I like to position myself in front of the large French doors in our kitchen, exposing myself to the many houses and overlooking windows that back straight on to ours. I close my eyes, spread my legs, and start to rub up and down over my slit, which is now very juicy and starting to drip. I put my legs high against the glass and continue to rub my slit and circle my clit, now and again inserting a finger or two into my shaven, dripping pussy. When I can take it no more I go to the fridge and take out a cold, half-peeled cucumber, go back to the window and start fucking it harder and harder until my pussy is throbbing and bucking with delight. Has anybody seen me this time? What would you do if you did?'

Let's Go Outside: If it was good enough for George Michael to sing about it, it should be good enough for us to try it. Those private parts between your legs have a distinct advantage over the boys', here, when it comes to outdoor self-play. It's so much easier for us to play outside than it is for our male counterparts.

I've been known to look at this as if I was on a covert operation, and I had to come at all costs. The one cost I wasn't prepared to endure was a night in the local lock-up for indecent exposure, so like all things when it comes to self-love use your common sense.

For the reason stated above, I like to take my self-pleasure sessions out into the woods on occasions. There is something both sexual and stimulating about being out in the open air. The idea of getting caught can turn out to be a bigger turn-on than you thought it might be. It might help if you wear a skirt and loose shirt. Find somewhere secluded and off the beaten track and begin to explore. You will likely find that bearing some, or all, of your naked flesh to the elements, you will get turned on very quickly. I often find that a session outdoors can be a lot shorter than those that take place indoors.

'I recently purchased an attachment for my garden hose with many different settings on it. I've always fantasized about masturbating outside, so I had to try it. I put the hose on the jet setting and directed it at my clit. It was so intense that I couldn't even keep it on my clit until I got extremely horny and was aching to cum. It was the most intense orgasm I ever had.'

Driving Me Crazy: I've heard many stories of people masturbating while driving and that is all well and good, but, to be honest, I wouldn't recommend it any more than I would texting or drinking and driving. If you feel the need to play with something other than your gearstick, I would strongly suggest you pull off the road first. Of course, if you are the passenger then all bets are off!

'It's probably really dangerous, but I like to masturbate while driving. I love it when strangers look into my windows. I start by playing with my nipples. I massage my breasts and gently pinch my nipples one at a time. I need to keep one hand on the wheel. I pull at them harder until I start to get little shivers going down my body, then I have to put my hand in my pants. I pull my pants down just enough to get my hand in, then I set the cruise control. I finger myself a couple times to get my pussy nice and wet. Then I lick my fingers and taste my sweet pussy juices. I circle my finger around my clit, not touching

it yet. The danger has made me so hot I know I'll explode as soon as I touch my clit. I go for it and roll it between two fingers really fast and start squirting almost immediately. Then I take a break and play with the little bit of hair I have down there before I do it again and again and again. By the time I get home my nice leather seat is soaked and I am very happy.'

Work It Baby: If you have your own office, then you are likely in luck and can spend some time when the need arises to take a break from work and do something, well, less boring instead. If, on the other hand, you work in an environment that is busy and filled with others, you may not be quite so lucky.

That said, self-pleasure, like all good sex, does not start in your nether regions, it all begins in your brain, and sometimes sexual stimulation can come from the seemingly strangest places. It could be that sexy customer, you know the one in the suit that fitted his slight, but extremely sexy body, to perfection. The guy or girl who prompted you to feel a sudden flush to overcome your cheeks as you served them. Take these moments and file them away for later, or if you really feel the need, the workplace toilet might just be your salvation.

If you do go down the public restroom, or even workplace, route, please be careful. Nothing spoils the mood quicker than being caught on the ummm 'job' and the words 'you are fired' are likely to illicit anything but feelings of euphoria.

'I have been at work now for two hours and already I am clenching my clit with my panties. I just came at my desk omg....I am soaking. I want to finger myself so bad. This morning I left for work and got the train. I have my skirt suit on and my tights are ripped at the crotch to make it easy to get to my pussy ...it takes an hour on the train so I usually finger myself under my coat and today was the

same. I am soaking all day. I have a stain on my seat at work. I cum
that often and soak the seat.

Now I am off to the washroom to finger the fuck out of my hole…'

Conclusion: When it comes to self-pleasure, nothing is off limits as long as you open your mind to the possibilities. I know, I keep saying this, but it's worth repeating. Please use your common sense when it comes to when, where, and how you decide to masturbate. That said, think outside the bed, and as you can see a whole new world of possibilities opens up.

CHAPTER 9

Advanced Masturbation Techniques

So by now, hopefully, you've either read chapter six and mastered at least some of the techniques that I mentioned there. If you haven't you might want to take a moment and go back and read it. Once that's done you are ready to try out what you might want to refer to as the 'ninja moves' of female masturbation. Okay, so they really aren't complicated, but there are times when I've been practicing masturbation that I swear I have resembled Luke Skywalker with his light saber, trying to channel the force. All that, of course, whilst trying to look totally cool as I wield said light saber in an attempt to find my often very elusive g-spot. I can only imagine it's not a pretty sight, but that's the great thing about masturbation at any level – you're the only one there, so looking silly is okay.

Unlike the techniques in chapter six these require some basic tools. Some of these tools require you to shell out a little, or a lot, of your hard-earned money, but others are items you may commonly find around your own house or apartment. I touched on sex toys in chapter six, but one thing I didn't cover there was how best to use a sex toy when masturbating. I felt that when it comes to sex toys, once you had the basics down it would be easier for you, as the reader, to digest their uses in a separate chapter and dunnuh here it is! Before we get into purchased sex toys, though, let's take a look at some of the more common household objects that both I and Clitical visitors have used throughout the years, because, let's face it, there are times when you just have an itch that needs to be scratched and you may not have the batteries, the budget, or the toy recharged at that precise moment in time – and I can tell you from experience, it sucks! So, without further ado, let's take a look at some advanced techniques.

Easy-Access Techniques
These techniques I named 'easy-access' as they require no special equipment other than objects that can generally be found around the home. They are also easy to implement and, in many cases, can lead to an orgasm as intense as any obtained from a store-brought toy.

It's In Your Jeans
Many women will tell you that they have found a great way to masturbate and all they require is to wear a pair of heavier jeans that, in turn, sport a thick seam at the crutch line. It's possible to simply sit and rock back and forth and create so much fiction between the seam and your vulva and clitoris. You can heighten this technique by placing your heel under your crotch and rocking back and forth. Many women find this a very enjoyable experience, whether or not they can reach orgasm this way. If, like me, orgasms from this technique are rare, it makes for some great undercover masturbation foreplay.

'I accidentally discovered this years ago when skin-tight designer jeans became popular. One day, when I was behind on laundry, I pulled on one of my tightest pairs of jeans with no underwear. Throughout the day, I realized that the crotch seam of the pants

120

pulled up deep into my cunt, stimulating my vulva. When I crossed my legs, the fabric would pull deep into my slit. Then as I walked, the seam would rub my cunt lips with every step. Delicious...'

Toothbrush Lover

Your humble electric toothbrush can become your best friend if you just give the relationship a chance. First things first, though, there are a couple of safety tips that I want to pass along before you dive head first into this affair. I strongly suggest that you purchase two toothbrushes, one for the lips in your head and the other for the lips between your legs. I've found that picking two different-colored handles can save a lot of confusion since, while toothbrushes are not prone to jealousy, there may be some cross-contamination if you get confused and use them on the wrong set of lips.

Once you have purchased your toothbrush, the fun can really begin. Find somewhere safe, where you won't be disturbed. Personally I like the bathroom and if you are at all worried about being found with your new best friend then this can be a great option. After all, who would suspect that you were intimate with your buzzing friend if you were discovered? Find a position that you are personally comfortable in. Maybe lying in the tub, sitting on the toilet, or lying in your bed – the choice is all yours. Whatever is most comfortable for you will work, and you may find yourself changing locations and positions over time – as your affair develops.

At this point I like to be naked, but I spend time removing my clothes while paying attention to my body as it is exposed. Sometimes I will tease myself, by using the brush to tease my nipples and breasts, stroking it across my skin as I travel down to my thighs. Sometimes I wait to turn the toothbrush on before I get to my thighs, sometimes not, depending on my mood. The sensations that are created vary, depending on whether the brush is turned on or off. Spend time experimenting to find what works for you.

By now I am generally wet between the thighs and my mind has begun to wander and create its own erotic images, the chances are yours will be, too. Now, slowly open your legs wider and begin to explore your vulva with the electric toothbrush. Feel free to use your free hand to part your outer and inner lips. Let yourself feel the sensations that your body creates as you explore every crack and crevice – and there are more of these than you might think hidden between your legs.

As you explore you will feel the sensations increase in your body. Pay careful attention to these sensations, where is your toothbrush placed when you receive the most pleasure? Spend the time getting to know your new lover, and you may just be surprised at the hours of pleasure you will receive for a little outlay. Couple that with the fact that your toothbrush will never say 'no', and you have a win-win situation here.

'If you don't have access to a vibrator, like me, use what you can find – an electric toothbrush! Turn it on and start at your clit, while also rotating the actual toothbrush head. Slowly (very slowly!) push it down to the opening of your vagina and stick it in. Within a minute or two, you'll have an awesome orgasm!'

'My favorite technique to use on myself is the electric toothbrush. I actually have one going on my clit as I type and it feels AMAZING! I am a college student and I have two roommates, so when I get the chance to masturbate I get really anxious. The excitement of them walking in on me or the next-door neighbors hearing me makes the experience soo much better.'

Shaver Favor

Just as the electric toothbrush can provide easily accessible vibrations, so can a battery-operated shaver or razor. Venus, as well as many male shaving companies, has a razor that features a vibration function and many women enjoy using this as a makeshift vibrator. With these types of shaver and whenever you are using them, common sense needs to come into play. Never use an electric razor with the blade attached as this obviously represents a huge safety risk. As with the electric toothbrush, if you find the vibrations are too intense you can add in a layer of material, like a pair of panties, to help deaden the power.

'I was in the shower one day feeling horny and suddenly noticed the amazing convenience of my Venus razor. I took the blade off so I didn't cut myself and began to rub the thick end up and down my clit before entering it into myself. The feeling was so amazing that I had to lie down on the floor of the shower because my legs were so weak. The handle of the razor has ribs so you don't drop it while you're shaving, but they're prefect for mind-blowing stimulation and the shape is absolutely perfect. I let the shower land on my clit and pumped the razor in and out with one hand while I played with my nipples with the other. I was able to have several orgasms – something I had not been able to do before.'

Pillow Talk

Pillows are not just for sleeping on any more; they can make for a useful masturbation tool. A lot of women find pleasure from humping their pillows as opposed to simply sleeping on them. All you need for this technique is one or two pillows that you then pile one on top of another between your thighs and you simply rock back and forth, or sideways, and create friction between the pillow and your clitoris. Many women can orgasm this way, and for many this is often their first introduction to masturbation.

'Stack three pillows up on top of each other on your floor or your bed. Then put down something to cover the pillow on top because you will get wet, I guarantee it. Get a t-shirt/washcloth/towel and roll it up hot-dog style. Get naked, at least your bottom half, and hump away. Feels soo good...'

'I actually found a new way to do it. Here is the story: I got super hot from these (Clitical stories) and I was so wet that my panties needed to come off. Needing to please my pink little clitty, I grabbed a pair of folded knee-high socks (the rougher the better.) I grabbed a stack of pillows (three or four for me) and I put on a fresh pair of underwear with the sock soaking up my sweet juices. I knelt above the stack of pillows humping and grinding smoothly. I started getting sooooo horny as I moaned my boyfriend's name. Ohhhhh yes. Uh huh. Fuck me. Fuck me. Baby harder. My bed shook intensely! Felt soooo good.'

Loving My Teddy

Many of us had soft toys and plushies when we were growing up, and some of us have never lost our love of the big furry bear or dog that sits on the end of the bed each night. The reasons for the strong feelings we have toward that bear or dog might not be quite why your mother thought it was, though, when she tried to get you to donate it to the nearest charity shop. For many women that soft toy was, to all intents and purposes, their first sexual partner. As many teenagers and older females will attest, plushies can be used to great effect when it comes to humping as a technique. A lot of women find that a large plushy with a rubber nose works well for this technique and they use the nose to tease their clitorises to the point of no return. A larger plushy can also be humped in the same way as a pillow can.

'Get a cuddly toy with a protruding nose and position your clit above the nose and hump the nose. When you feel you are about to *cum, stop, count to ten and start again and do this up to ten times and when you finally allow yourself to climax, the orgasm is mind-blowing electricity!'*

Veggie Fun

Many of us are familiar with the veggie sex jokes. You know, the ones that compare zucchinis, carrots, and cucumbers to dildos or penises. The strange truth is that in kitchens and bedrooms everywhere innocent vegetables are being shaped and carved into improvised sex toys. If you do use veggies to masturbate, I strongly urge you to wash and preferably peel your organic lover. It can be fun to take a large yellow squash and spend some time carving it into a shape that you think will please you. Personally I take the precaution of using a condom when I use veggies for self- pleasure and would strongly suggest you do the same. I would also not recommend using vegetables anally as they are not designed for the purpose and I really urge you not to use them this way. There is nothing gonna kill the mood faster than having to explain to a doctor how you have an entire carrot stuck in your ass, no matter which way you slice it!

'I have been masturbating since I was about 12 years old. I started out using my rolled-up sleeping bag. It served as a pillow between my legs. I would straddle it between my legs, with me on top, and pump away. Now that I am older, I have discovered that I really desire a more life-like experience when I masturbate. I have started to use cucumbers, bananas, and anything else shaped like a penis. I start off by getting my hands as cold as I can stand them by putting them in the freezer. Then I rub my tits with my cold hands, my nipples get super-hard and I rub them until my pussy gets wet and my clit starts to throb. Then I take my cucumber and stick it in my pussy. I then take a body pillow that I have and straddle it with the cucumber in me. I pump away until orgasm. This works great because the body pillow feels like a man is there and provides stimulation to my clit,

while giving me support for the cucumber to penetrate in and out. I really recommend this. I have used dildos before and gotten some pleasure, but the cucumbers really work for me.'

String of Pearls
Okay, so for this technique I'm in no way suggesting you borrow your grandma's real string of pearls, because that would probably be just plain wrong. What you can use instead is a set of mardi gras beads or even a beaded necklace. There are actually several ways in which you can use this innocent-looking device and the first is to simply use them to tease your vulva and clit. You can roll them, you can bunch them up, you can string them over your clit. You can even insert them into your vagina and pull them out slowly or quickly, as each movement will produce a different effect.

If you are feeling a little more adventurous you can use these same beads for anal masturbation, but there are a couple of safety checks you should always make first. Check the strength of the beads; try tearing them apart with your bare hands. If they spill out now, then you can imagine what would have happened had you inserted them somewhere else first. I strongly suggest you wash all improvised sex toys before you use them, or at least give them a spritz with a decent anti-bacterial sex-toy cleaner if possible.

'Hello! I have discovered a technique that makes my pussy ache to be licked and fucked by you sexy ladies! In the morning, before my classes begin, as I'm getting dressed, I slip a set of long beads in between my pussy lips. With half of the rest, I tuck it around my bra, to be secure, and the other half I lube up and put in my tight asshole. Throughout the day the beads rub my little clit as my ass is filled. This leaves me horny and my pussy throbbing the entire day. Sometimes I orgasm if I move around a lot during the day and I have to hide my moans from my professors! Personally, I like it better if I

126

don't because I can't wait to get home and fuck my dripping pussy. This method is well worth a try! Happy humping.'

Hairbrush Fun

A simple hairbrush can provide you with some new masturbation strokes – with a little imagination. Like store-brought sex toys hairbrushes come in a variety of shapes, sizes, colors, and shapes. They also have different strengths and thicknesses when it comes to bristles. Many Clitical visitors have reported using the handle of their hairbrush to either insert into their vagina or tease their vulva and clit. Others have used the business end of a clean brush, or at least I hope it's clean, to pet and tease their clits and vulvas. You can also use the back of the brush to gently spank yourself or run the bristle end of the brush over your entire body before allowing it to get anywhere near your nether regions. If this is your first time trying either of these techniques, I suggest you take it slowly until you figure out what works for you.

'I tried this technique last night, so much fun! Take something you want to fuck yourself with. I used a hairbrush handle. Stick the brush part in between your mattresses or couch cushions. Get your pussy wet and get on all-fours, back your wet pussy up on to the handle and fuck yourself till you cum.'

Write it Down

Sharpies or any other type of fat marker can make for a great improvised sex toy as long as you remember it's actually a pen and full of ink. Without wishing to state what should be obvious here, ink and vaginas do not mix and if you choose to use a sharpie or marker for penetration please use the end without the cap. A marker that still has the cap on can be used to write all manner of invisible messages on your body, as you work your way down to your vulva. It can be used to tease your clitoris and then be inserted into your vagina if you so wish.

'First undress completely. Start by rubbing your breast softly, then rub every part of your body. With a marker, start trapping your clit. It feel so good! And if you want, you can also insert it into your vagina. Just make sure it's clean! Have fun!'

50 Shades of Blind

It's a strange thing, but by taking away at least one of your senses, you can find that you will heighten the four that still remain. For this technique you will need something to use as a blindfold. I like to use my partner's silk tie, but that's just me. I'm sure there are plenty of suitable options in your closet if you care to look.

Now take your blindfold, and well, blindfold yourself, making sure that you truly can't see. Then start to touch your body. You can even be fully clothed when you start this technique, and, of course, naked or partly clothed will work as well. The point is that you will discover different sensations now that you can't see what you are doing. I've had some great orgasms this way, and it comes highly recommended as it allows you to concentrate on feeling the actual touch rather than on what you might look like.

'I just had one of the most amazing orgasms of my life and I would like to share it with you lovelies. In one word – blindfold. Pretty simple, hmm? I have found that when I'm a bit horny, I casually rub my fingers around my breasts and around my legs and collarbone, giving me goosebumps. Then I will strip down naked, the exposure heightening the feeling. I'll gently begin rubbing the outside of my pussy and slowly circle around my small clit. When I begin to get really excited, I take my sleep mask and put it on my eyes. Just cutting off that one sense will jump-start everything else – especially touch. I can more easily focus on where my fingers move, making my fantasies become more real. This simple technique made me lose control when I came, grinding into my fingers and making me shake and lose my breath. It's a surreal experience I suggest you try.'

Maxi Pads

Many women enjoy the feeling of riding a maxi pad, the type designed for periods as opposed to masturbation. The idea is a simple one. Just place the pad between your legs and ride away. Adding some friction in the shape of the edge of the bathtub can add another dimension to this version of humping.

'The first orgasm I ever had was during one of my early menstrual periods. I had been playing with myself for a year and got little thrills, but that was it. While baby-sitting two pre-schoolers we were playing with a plastic, ride-on chicken. I rode it and my pad was in great position so that as I rolled back and forth it rubbed me just right and I could not stop. The boys were transfixed and I found out what an orgasm was supposed to be. Although I switched, against my mother's wishes, to tampons soon after, I found other situations where rocking the pad could do the same thing. My only public orgasm was in history class as I rocked and rubbed on one of those old single- arm desk chairs. As I write this, I am wearing a pad and enjoying the motion on my desk chair.'

Candlelit Dinner for One

Candles may seem like the obvious candidate for a makeshift dildo, but the truth is that it's not easy finding the right fit. Most candles on the market are either too thin or too thick for most women to use at least comfortably. I've heard and read lots of techniques that suggest that candles can make great anal masturbation bedfellows, and I'll be honest, I cringe at the thought. Candles do not come with a flared base, and your sphincter muscle that is located in your butt is a lot stronger than you might think it is. It's more than capable of acting like a black hole and anything that you put in there that does not have a flared base to stop it is likely to disappear into said black hole. At that point, the only person who is likely to retrieve your candle is a doctor, and that's not fun for anyone.

I'm not saying you can't use a candle for some improvised fun, by any means. Just don't put it up your butt, okay? What you can use the common household candle for, and to good effect, is to tease your clit. Simply place the candle between your thighs and start to roll it back and forth. It may take a few tries to find a rhythm that works for you and, as always, you may not find you enjoy this method at all. If you do, you can experiment further by tapping the candle over your clit and, if you are feeling adventurous, why not try inserting it into your vagina. If you do go the insertion route, I strongly suggest that you use a condom, because while you might not get an STD as your candle-lover lights your fire, it is possible he is harboring some harmful bacteria, and safe sex is always the best sex, whether you are alone or partnered.

'Try this! While you're wearing super-silky short swimwear (the kind that you wear to the beach that look like super-short shorts but aren't) put either candles or highlighters, or both, if you're greedy, depends on how much you wanna masturbate (highlighters are the best!) in the freezer and wait for about 30 minutes till they're somewhat cold. Then sit on the edge of a computer chair and put the cold candle/highlighter in between your legs and move around in a circular motion. You can close (tighten) and open (relax) your legs while you're doing this. It feels great and you're in orgasm heaven in no time! Enjoy!'

Cell it to Me
Today's smart phones are very smart, in fact they are smart enough to help you masturbate, if only you would let them. Most smart phones, and even the older flip phones, have a vibration feature and you can put this to good use when it comes to masturbation. Simply ask a friend to call, place the phone on vibrate and between your thighs. If nothing else, it will likely bring a smile to your face and brighten your day. Who knows? It might bring you to orgasm if they call you enough to annoy you.

130

'I haven't posted in a while, but I had to post this. So I've been sexually frustrated as the old things I usually do won't work! Well, I was on my phone looking at some new free apps and came across a vibrating app. It looked normal and I always wanted to see why it was so popular. I hit gold! I downloaded it and checked it out, to find that it was a sexual vibe app! Well, obviously I had to try it! So that night I was in my panties and big t-shirt, lying down to watch some hot, lesbian porn: one tied up, the other fucking her brains out. Just to get myself wet and super horny. I turned off my lights, took off my panties, and hiked my shirt over my tits so I could play with 'em when I played my phone. I put my phone right on top of my clit and put it to level three of five. Oh god, it was heaven! Then I got into an angle sitting up to face my mirror, and after I turned the lights back on and pushed my phone hard on my clit, going to the fifth level, I watched as I rode my phone, watching my sheets stain with my overwhelmed hot juices!'

Ice, Ice Baby

This technique could, and maybe should, have gone into the water techniques section here, but I like to think it of sensation play. Ice and all its humble incarnations, such as popsicles, can be put to great use when it comes to masturbating. Try taking an ice cube or two and spend some time exploring your body. Start with your breasts, and if you are feeling adventurous, it's fun to do this in front of a full-length mirror. Watch the way your nipples react to the coolness of the ice as it begins to melt on your skin. Now move down your body, enjoying the sensations as you near your vulva. Some women find that ice is too cold a sensation for them and that's fine. Masturbation is about finding what works for you and your body, after all. If you do find the sensations pleasurable, you could place an ice cube or two in your vagina and enjoy the sensation of being full. You can also try all of these things with a homemade popsicle. To make your own simply take a popsicle mold, which can be purchased in most stores, and add just plain water, place in freezer and wait for a few hours. Many molds will make 6 of these at once and as one melts another is always handy.

Another way to use ice for masturbation is to take a long balloon and fill it with water until it fits the shape that you think will work for you. Now place the balloon in the fridge or freezer and wait a while. You can start with a completely frozen balloon if you like, or a semi-hard one. Now try the above technique with the balloon and experiment.

'Recently, I discovered a new technique that sends me into repeated shivering orgasms. I have a small plastic bag filled with ice, which kind of comes to a point on one end. I first start by rubbing over my nipples, and then slowly slide it down the front of my stomach. I tease myself by rubbing it in circles right outside my mound, and then slowly began to push it into my clit. Now, I lie down on my stomach and wiggle around until the ice hits just the right spot. I pump up and down on the ice chunk, until the feeling is so intense that I can no longer take it. The ice is so cold at first, but that just adds to the pleasure!'

Make-Up Sex
No, I'm not talking about making up after an argument with your partner or lover here. I'm referring to the almighty makeup brush. As with the hairbrush it can be used to great effect when it comes to masturbation, but unlike its larger counterpart, I would not recommend placing it in your vagina.

Spend some time brushing your entire body, before you attempt to touch your clitoris with the tip of the brush. Vary your strokes and pressure and discover what works best for you.

You can take this technique to an entirely new level by simply using the brush to draw the alphabet on your vulva. The result of this technique is that it can feel like a partner is giving you oral sex, and on occasion an orgasm has been known to ensue. Of course, you are not limited to just the alphabet, the sky is the limit here.

'*This technique can makes my pussy wet just thinking about it. First you take a small makeup brush, the ones used for applying eye shadow. Then you lie on the bathroom floor (I find the cold tiles of the bathroom a lot more sensual). Slowly use the brush around your nipples and slowly make your way down to your pussy. Gently make small circles with the brush directly on your clit, almost as if you're painting. You can feel your body rising and your pussy getting wetter and wetter, but don't be tempted to finish yourself off quickly. I'm doing it now in front of the computer, and I'm trying so hard not to give in to the temptations of my fingers. I'm slowly beginning to feel my body rise and shake...*'

Suck It Up
There are women who love to play with the vacuum cleaner and use the suction action of the hose to achieve orgasm. Whilst there is nothing wrong with this technique, remember that most vacuums are extremely powerful and if you do try this technique, I would strongly recommend putting a barrier between your delicate skin and the hose. This could be something as simple as keeping your panties on as you play or placing a towel over your vulva before playing.

'*I am always looking for something to get me off. So I decided to try the hose on the vacuum cleaner. OMG! I tell you. First, I lubed my clit up real nice. I placed the hose on my clit (be careful not to place it on your vagina entrance. I turned on the vacuum cleaner and moved the hose around. I came in less than five minutes.*'

Balls In
For this technique I enjoy the simple tennis ball, but you can try

it with any ball that feels comfortable for you. I find a hard ball with the fuzzy surface provides a great way to please yourself. Place the ball between your legs. This will work especially well if you lie on your stomach and allow the bed to act as a platform to hold the ball. Squeeze your legs tightly together and cross them at the ankles. Make sure that the ball is placed against your clitoris. Move back and forth on the bed in an up-and-down motion.

'When I am horny, I put one of those stress balls in a woolly sock and put it down my panties. I then lie on my back minus my bra, of course, and have one hand playing with my nipples while the other rubs at the mound in my knickers. I usually come fairly quickly as the gentle rubbing sets my clit on fire.'

Conclusion:
As I said at the beginning of this chapter, these techniques are by far the most popular that have been submitted to Clitical over the years and require little to no expense as many of the tools mentioned are common household items that most people will already own.

A few words of caution here. Just because it looks like a great masturbation tool, does not mean it is a good idea. If you are in doubt over an object's safety, my advice is please don't go there. There are many emergency-room doctors and nurses that will attest to the fact that putting a light bulb or glass bottle into your horny and gaping vagina is never a good idea, for example. Please see chapter eleven for more specific details.

CHAPTER 10

Toys, Lubes, and Other Things You Never Learned About in Sex Ed.

When I began writing this book, I knew I wanted to dedicate a chapter to sex toys and enhancers, but I also knew that this is a subject that requires its own book. It's such a big topic that all I can do is point you in the right direction and hopefully make your buying experience easier and more beneficial.

The truth is, there is an entire industry built on the belief that masturbation is good for you. That industry is aptly often called the 'pleasure industry' and whilst it has any amount of different facets, the one we are interested in, for the most part, is the one that deals with sex toys and enhancers.

Who Needs a Sex Toy?
There are no hard-and-fast rules when it comes to sex toys and who might need one. The simple truth is that many women have lived fulfilling lives without ever owning a vibrator, dildo, or any other type of sexual enhancer, and there is nothing wrong with that whatsoever. Owning a vibe should not be seen as some kind of rite of passage into womanhood, any more than not owning

one makes you less of a woman.

Of course, as sex toys have become more mainstream, thanks to programs like *Sex in the City*, which did more for rabbit vibrator sales than any rabbit has ever done for carrot sales, owning a vibrator is no longer considered to be something that belongs in the realms of risqué. In fact, the opposite is often true, and the reason for this is simple, sex toys are fun!

One of the reasons that Betty Dodson recommended that every women owned her own vibrator some 30 or so years ago was because not only are they fun, they take the hard work out of orgasm, for the most part. If you have never experienced an orgasm by your own hand, so to speak, a vibrator can be a great aid to your goal. Remember when we took our trip back in history, the part about why vibrators were invented, in order to help out poor doctors whose arms were tired and fingers sore from manipulating women to orgasm, well guess what, they are still good for that purpose today. I would add that the designs have, for the most part, gotten a lot better than the older electric massager styles, but the principal uses are still the same. Get me off, and make it quick.

What confuses most first-time sex-toy users is simply the vast selection of toys that is now available to virtually everyone over the age of 18. The good thing is, sex toys no longer have the same stigma that they had when I was first learning about them. Even 15 years ago, when I began reviewing them for Clitical, I rarely told anyone what I did, for fear of rejection. Now I think it's fair to say that owning at least one sex toy when you are old enough is a lot more acceptable, and in some ways, expected.

Where to Buy Your First, or Twenty-First, Sex Toy?
Thirty years ago, when I first became interested in sex toys, or sex in general, to be honest, there was little to no information

on the subject, and, if the truth be told, sex toys were awful. For the most part, a vibrator consisted of little more than a molded piece of hard plastic that resembled, and I use the word loosely, a penis shape. If you were lucky, they had more than one speed, but the most I'd ever seen was three. The only place you could purchase them were the seedy sex emporia, which were generally run by men and, like the material they contained, catered to men. The only women you generally saw entering or leaving were ones who were 'working'.

Fortunately over the last 30 years things have changed a great deal in the pleasure industry, and we began to see the emergence of the sex-toy industry as we know it now. The revolution began when sex became more of a mainstream experience for many women. Suddenly an orgasm was something we had to have, because we had read about it in *Cosmo* or any of the other female magazines that suddenly discovered that sex sells. Like many women of the time, my first foray into the world of sex toys was via an Ann Summers toy party. If you've never been to a sex-toy party they can make for a real fun evening. The basic premise is to gather a group of female friends, invite them to your house, ply them with wine, and let the company's hostess explain the latest and greatest sex toys, which were designed to give your love life a boost. We knew what they were for, but so many of us back then just assumed they were for bringing into partnered sex, which is strange looking back on it now. This was in part because, as we have discussed before, masturbation was not something that was ever discussed, even amongst close friends. We would all talk about our latest sexual exploits, of course, all giggle as the new girl on the block declared she was no longer a virgin, but never would we talk about being solo.

As sex-toy parties grew in popularity, so did the sex-toy industry. Companies began to cater to the needs of their clients, as opposed to just pushing out low-quality products that in many cases got the job done, but as we will see later, not necessarily in the safest way.

Shop My Way
The good news is that, thanks to Bill Gates, we now have the Internet and this has opened up an entire world of sex and sex toys, to the average Internet-user. A quick search on Google for sex-toy stores will yield you a staggering 3,180,000 results. Obviously, not all are relevant to you, but you get the idea. No longer are you limited to the local sex-toy store or your friend's party, you can now order worldwide, but this in itself can lead to problems. Which store do I choose? Which product will work best for me? How do choose, period?

If you are brand-new to the sex-toy world, I would seriously consider finding a female-friendly sex-toy store in your area and taking a trip over there. I live, by many standards, in the boonies, and my nearest sex-toy store is an hour's drive away, but I make the trip a couple of times a year and stock up. The advantage of these female- owned stores are threefold. The staff knows the products and which questions to ask you so that they can provide you with the right toy. You can touch, feel, and in some cases turn on, the toy in question. You are in an environment that does not judge. When I decide to visit my nearest store, I just make it a day trip and have fun when I reach my destination. Of course there are the 'adult' stores that many areas have and although my first choice would be to take a road trip to a more female-orientated store, these adult stores are not what they used to be when I was growing up. They do, however, tend to have less-knowledgeable staff and you are likely to find fewer quality toys than you would by driving a little further.

The other option is to simply hop on the Internet and find what you are looking for. Of course, this would likely be easier if you already knew what that was. Again you are likely to be bombarded with stores, so it pays to do some research and ask around, either between your friends or there are many respectable sex-toy bloggers out there who are more than happy to point you in the right direction. There is also a list of sex- toy stores that I have personally used and recommend within the resource section at the back of this book.

So you've decided where you are going to buy from, and now the only decision you should be faced with is which toy to purchase. It can be a little more complicated than that, but below you will find some pointers to help you make that very important, and sometimes costly, decision.

Stimulate Me the Right Way
Part of your research into what type of stimulation you enjoy should be a natural part of your masturbation routine. If all you need is to rub your clit and the magical orgasm genie appears, then you are in good stead as you already have your answer and all you need is a good clitoral-stimulation toy.

If, however, you are like many women and require a little more magic, perhaps in the form of some penetration, you may be better off looking for what I refer to as the dual-purpose toy; one that will allow you some penetration whilst still giving you some clitoral sensation. The most famous of these types of toys are the rabbit, which thanks in part to its appearance in *Sex in the City*, has become the most well known of the sex-toy types. Now, I will tell you that not all rabbits or sex toys in general are built the same and a rabbit is not always the prescription that your vulva and vagina were looking for. There are so many variations of the rabbit vibe now that even this basic toy can get confusing. Some have beads that rotate, some are made of plastic, some are made of silicone, while others have bells, whistles, and everything in between.

Another consideration you should take into account is where are you are most likely to use your toy. If you are a bathroom masturbator then you might well want to choose a waterproof toy, for obvious reasons. There are toys that are splashproof and it's worth noting here that these will likely not survive a trip into the shower. Another important consideration is the source from which the toy will get its power and the reasons for this consideration are not quite as straightforward as you might think.

Battery Versus Power Tools

Battery-powered toys are great for many occasions and they can provide some pretty powerful vibrations. They are often amongst the more discreet sex toy, but don't let that fool you. My first-ever foray into sex toys involved a little silver bullet vibe and it all but blew my socks off. Size should be a consideration, of course, but it should not be your only one. The downside of a battery-operated sex toy is that it requires, well, batteries, and this requires an extra purchase. It can also be annoying when your toy turns up in the mail and you have every type of battery in your house, apart from the type you need for this one particular toy, and yes, this has happened to me before.

Power tools are becoming more and more popular when it comes to the world of sex toys, and I'm not talking drills, saws, or nail guns here. Power tools are the type of toy that requires a wall outlet in order to run them. The downside of this type of sex toy is that unless you have an outlet close to the bed or wherever else you decide to play, they can be somewhat limiting. Also anything that requires plugging into an outlet during use should never be used in the bathroom and especially not the bath! Sounds obvious, but I'm willing to bet there are more than a few people who have had more of an electrifying experience than they were expecting. The upside of power toys is that because they get their juice directly from the power socket, they tend to be, well, more powerful, hence the name.

There is a way now, thanks to technology, that you can have the best of both worlds, though. Many of the more powerful toys now come with a rechargeable option and a charging cord that allows the user to have their cake and eat it, so to speak. These types of toys are generally more powerful than their battery-operated counterparts and because they do not need to be plugged in during use they can be used just about anywhere once fully charged. With that said, you should always check that a toy is waterproof before you attempt to use it in the tub or shower as not all toys are created equal.

Materials Are Us
As I touched on before, the choice of material that your sex toys are made from should definitely factor in to your decisions here. Below is a list of the more common types of toy materials available and each of their pros and cons.

Glass
Many people shy away from glass sex toys as they fear that they will break, but this, for the most part, is not true. Most glass toys are made from the same type of glass that is used to construct Pyrex bowls. Think about it. When was the last time you broke a Pyrex bowl? Of course, if you drop your glass toys on a granite floor tile, it may well splinter and be rendered unusable from a safety standpoint, but I have more than a few glass toys and all have stood the test of time.

Pros: Glass is inflexible, so if you like a hard, stiff penetration, the chances are you will enjoy glass-toy play. Often because of this inflexibility many women report that finding their g-spot is easier with glass than other types of material.

Simply put, they are beautiful. In fact they are so beautiful I have them on open display in the Clitical home office.

Glass lends itself very well to temperature play. Place it in the fridge for a chilly experience or a bowl of hot water to warm up your masturbation experience.

Glass is by nature non-porous so it's hard, as long as you are cleaning your toys properly, for them to harbor bacteria.

Cons: Can break or splinter if dropped on a very hard surface.

Require a considerable investment, as the better-quality glass toys, like those that come from the company Fucking Sculptures, are not cheap, but in my estimation are well worth the cash as you are not just buying a sex toy but a work of art.

Silicone
Since its emergence onto the toy market, silicone has become the most popular of all the toy materials. Silicone comes with something of a caveat, though, as not all silicone is created equally. Some is blended with other materials and although it will feel like the real deal, it can be something of a wolf in sheep's clothing. That said, there are several reasons why silicone has gained in popularity as a sex-toy material.

Pros: Silicone feels soft and in many ways lifelike, it's hypoallergenic and warms up quickly to body temperature.

It's non-porous, which makes it easy to clean and it can, in fact, be boiled.

Durable and long-lasting.

Cons:

Pure silicone sex toys can be a little more pricey than their counterparts,

As a general rule, it's not a good idea to use a silicone toy with a silicone lubricant. They do not play well together and you run the risk of damaging your expensive toy, so stick to your favorite water-based lube to be on the safe side.

Jelly

It's rare that I will tell anyone to steer clear of any sex-toy material, but the one exception to that rule, would be jelly sex toys. The material itself is made from a concoction of PVC and rubber and is, in many cases, instantly recognizable by its distinctive odor, which is very chemical in nature. Back in the days when the sex-toy market was beginning to blossom, many manufacturers created toys out of jelly and the reasons were simple. They were cheap to manufacture and the consumer was not as well informed as they hopefully are today. Most manufacturers are no longer producing jelly toys because of the health risks that have been associated with them. Jelly is porous by nature and therefore cannot be cleaned properly, and it has been known to create some nasty bacterial infections. As if that was not enough, they are also often made with phthalates, a substance that softens the rubber and allows it to be more flexible. Phthalates are believed to come with some health concerns and, again, are being phased out in the adult industry.

Pros: There are none and I would strongly advise you not to waste your money on jelly toys.

Cons: Jelly toys period! They are porous, can harbor bacteria and for that reason alone should never be used without a condom.

Rubber
You can often find simple latex rubber being used in the production of dildos as they produce a much, ummm, stiffer dildo than silicone or jelly. They tend to be very firm, in fact, and are also quite lifelike. So if you like your dildos on the more realistic side, rubber is not a bad choice. That is, unless you happen to be sensitive to latex – and many women are. The upside of a rubber dildo is that they tend to be cheaper than their silicone counterparts, but are porous, so I would recommend using a condom in conjunction with them.

Pros: Cheaper than silicone.

Lifelike feel and more rigid than many toys on the market.

Cons: Rubber is porous by nature and should always be used with a condom where possible.

People with latex allergies should avoid it at all cost.

TPR & TPE Sex Toys
TPR (thermoplastic rubber) and TPE (thermoplastic elastomer) material are virtually indistinguishable from one another. Both are considered Thermoplastic Elastomers, a material that is *often* phthalate-free. Be warned, though, both materials are porous and it's always a good idea to use them in conjunction with a condom because of this.

Additionally, this material is generally lightweight and durable. TPR is environmentally safe and made of 100 per cent non-poisonous raw material, which is preferable for most women and men. Compared to silicone and pure elastomer, TPR is slightly less impressive – though TPR sex toys are generally inexpensive in comparison to their two counterparts. In comparison to jelly rubber, TPR is the better material, if slightly more expensive.

Pros: Lightweight and flexible
Less expensive than many other toys on the market.

Cons: May contain phthalates. Please be sure to check the descriptions on the packaging or website before you decide to buy.

Porous, so using a condom with these toys is preferable.

Hard Plastic
In general, hard plastic toys are non-porous and therefore are easy to clean. Hard plastic is also phthalate-free. There is very little give in this type of material and if you prefer a sex toy that is rigid this can be a great choice.

Pros: As I said, if you like your toys on the more rigid side, hard plastic can provide this.

Easy to clean due to it not being porous.
Phthalate-free, which is always a plus.
Tends to be one of the cheaper toy types and materials.

Cons: Some of these toys can have sharp edges due to the molding process and should be checked for these before use. If you find any, there is a simple solution. All you need do is take a nail file and file down the sharper edges until they are smooth.

Metal
High-quality metal toys are a great material, especially if you enjoy a less-rigid feel when you are playing with toys. Metal toys are 100 per cent phthalate-free and are very smooth. I would not recommend a painted metal toy, as these can be prone to flaking

and nobody wants that in their most sensitive places.

Pros: Rigid simply because they are metal and if this is a type of stimulation you like then metal can be worth trying.

100 per cent phthalate-free.

Very smooth

Easy to clean because they are non-porous.

Cons:
Painted metal toys can flake and are best avoided.

Softskin and Cyberskin Sex Toys

Cyberskin and Softskin are both materials that make for soft, supple, and skin-like material. Thanks, in no small part, to the fact that toys made from either substance have an extremely realistic feel, they have over the past few years grown in popularity. The main difference between the two materials is that whilst Cyberskin is phthalate-free, Softskin is not, so Cyberskin is considered the better choice of the two materials. It's also worth noting that both types are porous and can be hard to clean because of this.

Pros: Extremely realistic in both coloring and feel. If you are looking for something that not only resembles a real penis but feels like one this might be a great choice for you.

Cyberskin is phthalate-free whilst Softskin is not.

Cons: Very hard to clean and sterilize because they are both porous in nature.

Only water-based lubricant should be used with both of these materials.

It's worth noting here, the makers of Cyberskin and Softskin toys do not share all of the ingredients that are used in the making of these toys. Due to this it's impossible to rule out the possibility of some latex being used in the material, so people with latex allergies may want to ask before they buy.

As you can see, there is a lot of choice when it comes to sex-toy materials, and being informed about the pros and cons of each is a great way to avoid any pitfalls that are so common for especially first-time buyers.

Bang For Your Buck

You've worked hard for your money and you are investing some of it in a toy that will help you achieve an orgasm. Many first-time buyers will purchase the cheapest toy they can find, in the mistaken belief that any toy will do – as they all do the same thing. If this were true, the person who invented those plastic penises I was so familiar with during my teen years would be one rich dude by now. This is where research becomes your first port of call and by doing your research you can determine the best toy type and material for you. Once you have decided on a material for your new toy, you will want to decide exactly what kind of toy is right for you. As I discussed before, there is a huge selection available to you, but this can be broken down into easy categories, which makes it easier for you to decide.

Store-Brought Sex Toys

There are so many toys on the market today that you could be forgiven for thinking you have no idea where to start, let alone how to decide which toy is right for you, so let's start by taking a tour of the four basic types of toys out there and their uses:

Dildos

Dildos have been around since the dawn of mankind, or to be more accurate, womankind. If for no other reason, I believe that dildos deserve some serious respect and yet they are often seen as the 'poor woman's dick', you know, the poor woman who can't get a real penis to do the horizontal tango with her. I think that's a shame and it's time we stopped thinking like that as a society and gave dildos the respect they deserve. Back in the bad old days, before sex toys and dildos came out from under a rock, dildos were made to resemble the male penis, but times they are a-changing. Nowadays dildos come in as many shapes, colors, and designs as you can think of –and a few I bet you haven't yet. Whilst there are many dildos that attempt to look, and even feel, like the real penis deal, be that a dolphin or a man's penis (yes, there are a several companies out there that produce dildos of the more exotic kind – from aliens to realistic animal penises), there are also plenty of dildos that do not look anything like the real deal. But, the truth is, they are all designed to do one thing: fill your vagina. Yes Virginia, penetration is most definitely the name of the game when it comes to dildos. With that in mind, let's take a look at some of the things you might want to consider when choosing which of these dildos might be right for you.

Do You Want a Dildo that Looks Like a Penis or Would You Prefer a Less-Realistic Type?

This is, of course, all about preference, but it is something you should consider before you start looking. Some of the realistic dildos are just that, realistic – in both color and feel. With techno-logical breakthroughs in the adult industry there are many dildos that offer close to the real thing. Real Feel and Cyberskin have both revolutionized the industry in this respect. If you prefer something that is a little less realistic, I would recommend you take a look at the plethora of glass dildos that are filling the market these days. Not only are these functional, many are stunningly beautiful and can be displayed for the world to see, without them having any idea what you are going to be using them for later.

How Much Are You Willing to Spend?

There are dildos on the market that cost as little as $15 and some that go to the other end of the spectrum and cost over $300. In general with a dildo, as any other sex toy, you get what you pay for and the more of your hard-earned cash you are willing to spend the better the product. That's not to say that a great dildo can't be had for a lesser price by any means, it pays to shop around, though, if you can. Glass toys, such as those produced by 'Fucking Sculptures', can run as some of the more expensive, but what you are buying is basically functional art when you buy one of their dildos.

What Kind Of Materials Do You Enjoy?

There are as many kinds of dildos out there and choice of material is, as with everything else, something of a personal choice. There are dildos made from various materials that have a little give in them, whilst others, such as glass, are completely rigid. This is, once again, where masturbation can come in handy as a guide. If you enjoy masturbating with a cucumber, for example, you might want to consider a material such as silicone, which will allow you some give. If, on the other hand, you prefer a sharpie pen, or hairbrush, handle a glass, wooden, or metal dildo might suit your needs better.

What Size (as in what width) Do You Prefer/Need?

When it comes to choosing the right size for you, masturbation can, again, make your decision easier. When it comes to size, many people consider this to mean length, but the width or circumference of a dildo or a vibe is something that is more important to consider. There is a huge difference between a one-inch dildo and a five-inch one, after all. This is where, if you can, go to your local female-friendly sex-toy store. I would strongly advise you to make that trip. It's hard to visualize a five-inch-wide dildo unless you are holding it in your hands. That said, if you really can't visualize it, take some common everyday objects like a coke can and a tape measure and, well, measure its circumference to give you a visual idea of what size you are looking at. Equally, if you have a favorite improvised sex-toy, measure its circumference to get an idea of the size that will work for you. I would generally advise that you choose a toy smaller than you think you need if this is your first-ever dildo, but again this is a personal choice.

What Shape and Texture do you Prefer?

Dildos come in a variety of shapes and textures. Some are smooth, whilst others have ridges and round knobs in strategic places that are designed to hit certain spots in your vagina. There is some debate as to whether these textures add to a female experience due to the fact that, in reality, only the first couple of inches of your vagina are actually sensitive.

When it comes to shape, the main consideration is whether or not you would like to reach your g-spot or not. Some women do not enjoy g-spot play, whereas others crave it. Again, as with all things sexual, this is about personal preference. If you do want to try, or know, that you love having your g-spot stimulated, then there are plenty of dildos that are designed to help you hit the right spot, so to speak.

Vibrators

Believe it or not the humble vibrator has been around in one form or another since 1869, when the first steam-powered vibrator was patented by an American doctor. It was hailed as a labor-saving medical device that would allow doctors and nurses to spend less time manipulating females to orgasm and it's been doing the job very well in various guises ever since. Nowadays vibes are, thankfully, no longer steam- powered, but the idea behind them is still the same as it was back then, to give women an orgasm and make it easier to achieve one.

Finding the right vibrator for you might seem like a daunting task, given that there are so many on the market nowadays. I would strongly suggest you either take a trip to a reputable sex-toy store, where it is possible to ask questions and in many cases pick up and feel the vibration, measure the sound, and generally chat to some knowledgeable sales staff before you make your choice.

If that is not something you can do, then I would strongly suggest you spend some time on the Internet and visit some of the sex-toy reviewers' blogs I have listed in the resource section at the back of this book. Bear in mind, what works for one person may not work for another, but sex-toy reviewers already know this and will take it into account when they write a review. Most will list important points, including the pros and cons of each toy they review and this can be an invaluable source for many.

When you start shopping for a vibe there are some questions you might want to ask yourself in order to help you figure out which one is right for you.

1: Which part of your body do you actually want to stimulate? Your clitoris, vagina, g-spot, or a combination of all three?
If you are already masturbating, the chances are you already have some idea as to what areas of your body you would like to try a vibrator on. Most reputable online stores can help you here as they often list vibes not only by type but also by body areas that the vibe is designed to be used on. For example, a clitoral vibe, as the name suggests, is best used on the clitoris.

2: Are you looking to buy just one vibrator or a variety?
The reasons it's worth asking yourself this question is that many vibes are designed to cover more than one type of stimulation. I like to call these dual-purpose vibes. The most commonly known of these types of vibe would be the rabbit, which was made

famous by *Sex in the City*. A rabbit vibe is designed to stimulate both your clitoris and vagina at the same time, although they can be used independently.

3: Do You Intend to Use the Vibrator for Penetration?

Not all vibes are meant to be inserted inside the vagina, so if you really enjoy penetration, this is something you might want to consider before you purchase.

4: What type of vibrations are you looking for?

Again, if you already masturbate, then you should have good idea what the answer to this question is. If it takes little more than a few light strokes of your clitoris to bring you to orgasm, you might consider the cheaper battery-operated vibes. If, on the other hand, you prefer a more intense vibration or heavy hand, then you may want to consider investing in an electric-powered, or rechargeable, vibrator. This type of vibe generally offers a much more powerful vibration than battery-operated counterparts.

5: Is Noise Something You Need to Consider?

If you share a room or house with roommates then you might want to take the noise level of a vibe into consideration before you make your purchase. This is something that sex-toy reviewers generally report on as part of their reviews.

6: Do You Enjoy Water Play?

The reason I ask is simple. If you enjoy masturbating in the shower tub, or even pool, a waterproof vibe is a must, for obvious reasons. A word of caution. There is a big difference between a waterproof and a splashproof vibe, with the first being designed to be fully submerged in water, whereas the splashproof type will only allow you to wash the vibe safely and I would not recommend taking it into the shower or tub.

7: Do You Travel a Lot?

If you do travel, do you intend to take your new friend with you? If you do, then you might want to consider things like travel locks, which many higher-quality vibes feature nowadays. These locks are designed to turn off the vibe and offer no possibility of starting up again once it is settled into your luggage or hand carry. There are also several smaller, discreet vibes on the market that are easy to disguise in your luggage if you are a little worried about it being discovered by airport security.

8: What Price Are You Prepared to Pay?

In general, the more expensive a toy is, the better the material it is constructed from. Also, rechargeable and electric toys are more expensive than their battery-operated counterparts. However, you may go through so many batteries during the lifespan of your battery-operated vibe that in the end the electric version will prove to be cheaper in the long run.

The above is by no means an exhaustive list and, once again, I urge you to take to the Internet, talk to your close friends, and think before you make that purchase. A little research now can avoid a lot of disappointment later, that's for sure.

Anal

Anal sex toys have become popular over the past few years as anal play has become more acceptable in society. When you play anally and, as we discussed before, playing anally when solo can bring a whole new sensation to the sexual arena. I strongly recommend not using found sex toys. There are a number of reasons for this. First your ass is designed to push stuff out of it, and we all know what stuff I'm talking about here. It is not designed to have stuff pushed into it, but if you do so, be aware that the strong muscles that allow you push stuff out of your body can, and will, work in reverse and suck it right into you. This is why anything that you may decide to put into your backside should always, always have a very flared base or, better still, be designed for the job at hand. Obviously the main purpose of your ass is to expel poop from your body. Poop is not user-friendly and can contain harmful bacteria, so using safety precautions when playing with anal toys is always a good idea. There are some women who enjoy an enema before they play anally. The enema is designed to flush out any poop that may be hiding in the lower sphincter muscles that form the anus and for some women it can be a sexually charged and satisfying experience. Personally I like anal toys that are made from silicone for a couple of reasons, the main one being that a good silicone anal toy can be boiled and sterilized. You can even use bleach as well. There is one other thing I would recommend if you do decided to try anal self-play and that is a good-quality lubricant. Unlike your vagina, your ass does not lubricate itself, and if you simply take a toy and try pushing up there, it's gonna hurt. Period. By allowing yourself time to get ready for the toy, and adding in some water-based or silicone-hybrid lube, you may find that anal play is something which, especially when used in combination with vagina or clitoral play, can make for a very pleasurable experience. There is a variety of anal toys on the market today, so let's begin by exploring some of these toys and their uses, shall we?

Butt Plugs

Butt plugs are basically dildos that are designed especially for use in your butt, as the name suggests. Anal plugs come in many different shapes and materials, but all have one important feature: a flared base. As I stated before, this is so they can't wriggle out of your grasp and require a trip to the ER. Some of the basic shapes of butt plugs are diamond, spiraled, and corkscrewed. Most begin with a narrow end and lead to the flared base. All are designed to be worn during masturbation or partner play and many women find wearing a butt plug whilst masturbating can lead to a very pleasurable experience. When you insert a butt plug, angle it upward toward the front of your body. It can also help to twist the plug slightly in order to get the widest part of the plug past your sphincter muscle.

Butt plugs can also be used for, what I like to call, masturbation foreplay. Many are designed to be worn for extended periods of time, and the feeling of fullness they create can make an afternoon in the office or the laundry more enjoyable and the anticipation of removing it can add a new dimension to your solo play.

There are butt plugs that are also designed to vibrate after they are placed in your anus and again can add a new dimension to anal solo play.

Anal Beads
Anal beads, as the name might suggest, consist of a string of beads that are designed to be fed into your anus and then removed either with one sharp tug or one at a time. Many anal beads feature what I like to call a 'graduated set'. In other words, they begin with a smaller or larger bead and graduate to the other end of the scale. Anal beads come in as many designs and materials as plugs and the ones I like to use the most are again made from silicone. This, again, is based on hygiene for me, but you can try the other materials that are out there for starters. There are some women who report that they have played anally with mardi gras beads. Whilst these types of beads are fine for vaginal play, anal play is not something I recommend as these beads and, more importantly, the string that cheaper beads are often threaded on to may break during play and would require a trip to the ER to remove the beads themselves. Personally, I would spend a few dollars more and purchase a toy designed for the purchase. Another issue with beads not specifically made for the job at hand is that they often have sharp edges that could scratch what is a delicate area of your body and, in turn, lead to infection.

Having said all of the above, anal beads can be real fun to experiment with. Make sure, as always, the beads and the outer opening of your anus are well lubricated and then begin to feed the beads upward and inward. This can be a little tricky to master, but once you figure out the right position for you, it becomes much easier. Some women prefer to pull the beads out as they reach orgasm through clitoral stimulation, whilst others find this too intense and either do it right before or after. Finding what works for you can prove to be a lot of fun, though. One other difference between anal beads and plugs is that beads are NOT designed to be left in the anus.

Whatever type of anal toy you purchase, you want to consider a few other issues. The most important of these decisions will be how large you think your plug or the largest bead on your bum necklace should be. My suggestion here is to be realistic. Whilst the biggest, widest butt plug might satisfy your ego, if this is your first foray into anal play it might not be your best choice.

Readers Techniques
'Very simple and honest… I love masturbating and always do whatever it takes to have the strongest orgasms possible! My best advice is to spend whatever it takes to buy the right sex toys. Try buying yourself a powerful two-speed vibrating massager, two extra-large soft-skin silicone dildos, water-based lube and one of those muscle simulators that shock you. Everything else is pretty obvious. lol.

Place one dildo in your vagina and the other in your ass, using plenty of lube on both. Place the muscle-stimulating pads between your legs and hold the massager on your clit till you can't take any more and cum. I always masturbate solo and usually with a porno on the TV. I sometimes play loud music and connect headphones to the TV, so nobody knows what I'm doing in my locked room. I've tried masturbating many different ways and nothing even compares to this. Hope you enjoy!'

'I like to use a "silver bullet" on my clit and a firm dildo at the same time. I have found that when I slide the dildo in and out, I push it against the bullet and it puts a sensational vibrating pressure against my clit (and it keeps the bullet from slipping out, freeing my other hand to pinch a nipple) I like to start out with the bullet on low and as I feel my orgasm building, I increase the speed…and pull my knees way back against my chest. With the in-and-out motion, I climax very hard.'

'I am 46 years old and have been masturbating since age 13. I have always been very sexually active (including three marriages and several live-in relationships), yet masturbation has always been a large part of my life. I have a 27-year-old live-in now, who was born way too late for his time and has actually taught me that solo sex is wonderful, not a thing to be hidden. My favorite technique involves "lots" of KY, a dildo, a little "rush" for the head (something wacky to smoke beforehand will put you in an even "hornier" mood!), and the good ol' reliable fingers. My technique involves ass fucking for the big part. I like to lie on the bed and have a porn movie on for added effect…also have a mirror propped between my legs to see what I'm doing…this gets me even more excited. I begin by rubbing my clit and putting a finger in the vagina. I also like to use clamps on my nipples (they can stand a lot because of insensitivity after a breast reduction). I get myself worked up, then lube up an eight-inch dildo with KY. This goes in the ass, which is much more exciting to me than a vibrator in the vagina. During these episodes I am hitting off a bottle of Rush, which really intensifies sex in any way. I fuck my ass hard with the left hand while rubbing horizontally across my clit with my right hand. I can hold off as long as I like and really have the most INTENSE orgasm ever because once I cum this way I am spent for at least an hour. (Just a little suggestion: prior to this an enema can be beneficial for "cleaner" results.) I think it's time I went to try out my "method".'

Lubricants: Slippery When Wet

If there is one thing that they never taught you in sex ed, but probably should have, it's this: diamonds are not a girl's best friend, but personal lubricants are.

If you think personal lubes are something that only older ladies and guys need, you might want to think again. Personal lubricants can not only make any masturbation experience more pleasurable, there are times when I think they are required. Today there is a seemingly overwhelming array of personal lubricants on the market. The lubricant market is, in fact, one of the most competitive markets within the pleasure industry. So where to start? I generally find it's always best to start at the beginning, so go grab a coffee, settle back in your comfy chair and we'll begin our crash course in personal lubricants.

Homemade Lubes

There are some people who have found that they can use common household oils and potions rather than spending a few bucks on manufactured lube. On the face of it this might sound like a great idea, but there are some health risks associated with this type of lube. So let's start by taking a look at the safety issues that can arise from concocting your own personal lubricants.

Many people love to use common household oils as a lubricant. I'm not talking WD40 here, but more the kind you find in the kitchen. Olive oil, coconut oil, and vegetable oil have all been popular choices that I have seen mentioned over the years. It's worth remembering that these oils are meant for eating and some people have allergies to oils such as peanut, so placing them on some of the most delicate skin on your body might not be the best idea ever.

They are also oil-based and oil and latex do not play well together.

Many times you will see me recommending the use of a condom whilst using a toy and as most condoms are made from latex, if you use an oil lube, you might as well not bother with the condom. The oils break down the fiber of the condom and over time the condom will lose the safe-sex effects that you are hoping to achieve.

Culinary oils are also designed for eating, not for use during sex and because of this can contain some impurities. Some products can cause irritations when they are applied to the skin and, to be honest, are best left in the kitchen, as they can produce some unwelcome side effects.

Manufactured Lubricants
Choosing the right lube for you

There are several factors that can play into your decision when it comes to choosing a lube. The first is that it should be made and used for your intended purpose. The second is that you should take into consideration the material a toy is made from. The best advice here is if you aren't sure, stick to the water-based variety as these are generally safe with all types of toy materials.

Another thing to take into consideration is the ingredients of each lubricant. These are almost always in plain view on either the packaging or on the lube container itself. By knowing what ingredients are in a product it's far easier to make an informed decision.

Nowadays there are many different types of lubes, including organic and vegan, both of which will, generally, have a shorter life span that those that contain more chemical components. It can also help you track down any ingredients that you might be sensitive to.

Lubes come in three basic types: water-based, silicone, and oil, and knowing which lube is right for the job at hand can save you both a lot of money and time, and, on occasion, a possible trip to the doctor.

Let's start by taking a look at the three types of lube and what jobs they perform best.

Water-Based Lubes
These are the most common of the lube groups and are the foundation for many lubricant companies, and for good reason. Unlike their silicone and oil counterparts they are pretty much safe on every toy material, perform well and are tried and tested as good substitutes for the other readily available water-based lube, more commonly known as human saliva. Whilst saliva can be used as a lubricant, it can also carry bacteria according to recent studies and is not formulated for the purpose for which you are using it. A good water-based lubricant is safe to use on all toy materials and can make masturbation a very pleasurable experience.

Pros: **Water-based lubes** are safe to use with condoms.

Safe with use on all sex toys, the cucumber covered with a condom will not object either.

Easy clean up. A simple wipe of a wet washcloth and you are good to go.

Cons: Water-based lubes can dry out quite quickly and many will take on a sticky feel. The good news is there is a simple fix for this. Simply place a spray bottle of water next to your bed and if you feel the lubricant begin to dry out, spritz your vulva and the lube will magically reactivate itself.

Water-based lubes suck for use with any kind of water play where you are submerged. I have had some success when using them in the shower, but there are better choices, to be honest.

Silicone-based lubes

As the name suggests, this type of lube comprises mainly silicone and has certain attributes that make it an excellent choice in certain situations. I love to use silicone-based lube if I am playing with toys in the tub. The silicone the lube contains is waterproof to a much greater degree than its water-based counterpart.

Pros:

Great for water-based play.

Like water-based lubes, silicone is safe to use with latex-based condoms.

Cons: Silicone toys and silicone lube do not play well together. I'm not a molecular chemist and I'm not even going to try and explain the science behind this. You will just have to take my word for it, and that of scientists around the world, that mixing the two can lead to some really squishy, gooey toys. Slippery as all hell. If you choose to use a silicone lube whilst in the tub, I strongly suggest you sit down. I learned this lesson the hard way when, during the midst of a very delightful orgasm, as I stood in the shower, I slipped on some errant silicone lube and fell backward into the tub!

Clean-up gets a little tougher with a silicone lube and requires the application of some soap and warm water in most cases.

Oil-Based Lubricants

As the name suggests, these lubes are constructed from an oil-based substance. Whilst this makes for a very durable and slippery lubrication, the downsides often outweigh the upsides of this type of lube.

Pros: Oil-based lubes feel sleek and are not easily absorbed by the skin, which means they require frequent reapplication.

Oil-based lubes make great external water-play partners. Please avoid placing them in your vagina or anus as they are almost impossible to remove and can, in some cases, cause infection.

Cons:

Oil and latex do not mix and therefore should not be used in conjunction with your protective condom. The oil will break down the condom and make it much weaker. It is the hardest of all the lubes to clean up. Oil and water do not mix and so some soap and water is required and even that is not guaranteed to remove this type of lube. It can cause stains on the bed sheets.

Conclusion:

Choosing a lube can seem like a daunting task, but by following the simple guidelines above you can take some of the angst out of the buying process. Many companies and firms now produce sample packs of lube that contain a variety of the range they carry. This can be an excellent starting point that allows you to explore the wonderful world of lubes without breaking the bank. I would recommend buying a personal lubricant as opposed to experimenting with home-made concoctions and I would definitely caution you to stay away from Vaseline and baby oils, as tempting as they might seem. By purchasing a product that is formulated specifically for the purpose of providing you with lubrication, you are on the safer end of the spectrum.

When it comes to choosing a sex toy, I strongly recommend visiting some of the sex bloggers that are listed in the resources section of this book. These are women who know their sex toys, often literally back to front. They can be a great place to discover tips, as well as keep up with current trends within an ever-evolving industry.

CHAPTER 11

Warnings AKA 'You Put What Where?'

Always Practice Safe Solo Sex

Normally when you read or think about 'safe sex' you'll think of it in terms of partnered sex and all too often solo sex is left out of the equation. Whilst it's true that it can be harder to get into trouble via solo sex, it's by no means impossible. Don't just take my word for it, though, ask any ER nurse or doctor – they all have stories to tell.

I've never been quite sure what the actual cause of this is, but over the years I've come to the conclusion that when humans get turned on and very horny, common sense seems to fly out of the window. Now, I'm not suggesting for a second that turned on equals stupid, but there are plenty of times when I've been reading though some of the techniques that have been offered up at Clitical that I have found myself questioning that basic assumption.

As I mentioned in chapter seven there is a wide variety of household objects that can be used in the pursuit of self-pleasure, but to be honest, just because you could use something, this doesn't

163

always mean that it's a good idea. Nothing cures a sudden bout of horniness quiet like a trip to the ER at 3am to remove that glass coke bottle that looked like such a great prospect earlier. There is now an entire television series devoted to the point where dumb and horny ideas collide, and plenty of ER doctors and nurses that will attest that this is one of the more common reasons why people end up in ER. By taking some simple precautions you can easily avoid that embarrassing trip or, worse still, being on TV or in the local newscast. So let's take a look at some of the more common ways that you can practice safe solo sex and avoid that trip.

I Love the Sound of Breaking Glass
Generally speaking, it's never a good idea to place anything made of glass inside your vagina or anus. The only exception to that rule would be if you were using a glass toy that was specially designed for the purpose. Glass toys are made from broscillate glass, which is known more commonly as Pyrex, but your average coke bottle is not and will often shatter. Another popular item with female masturbators seems to be glass light bulbs and whilst the shape might seem like fun and sexy, if the glass shatters whilst it is inside you it's anything but sexy.

Assing Around
Talking of your anus, whilst it can be fine and dandy to place things in your anus, there is one rule you should always follow, whether you are using a sex toy, candle, or anything else you found lying around the house. If it doesn't have a flared based or is not designed for the purpose, please don't do it. The reason for the flared base principle is simple. Your anus contains some mighty powerful muscles as well as a ton of nerve endings. Those muscles can work against you when it comes to penetration, as they will suck anything upward that you choose to stick in your anus. Having a flared flat base at the bottom of an object prevents this from happening.

Keep a Lid on It

Another popular choice for female masturbators is the humble bottle. Coke bottles seem to be high on the weapons-of-choice list when it comes to masturbation and if you choose to use any type of bottle, I urge you, for your own safety, to keep the lid on that bottle. Whilst the vacuum that not having the lid on produces might feel good, it can, and often will, produce the unwanted effect of not wanting to let go of said bottle when the vacuum inside yourself and the bottle has reached melting point. The same is true if you choose another favorite improved masturbation tool, the humble sharpie marker. In this case, I would advise that you don't place the tip into your vagina at all. Use the thinner part of the marker and always make sure the lid is properly secured before inserting.

Condoms Are Your Best Friend

So, we are, for the most part, well aware of the benefits of condoms when it comes to partnered sex, but they are often forgotten when it comes to solo adventures. Whilst it's true that it is very hard to get pregnant when you're by yourself, there are some situations that still call for a condom.

If you are using an unfamiliar sex toy that perhaps you borrowed from a friend, please be sure to place a condom over it. I'm not saying or condoning sex-toy sharing here, but I live in the real world and it happens.

If you are using a home-made or improvised toy, such as a vegetable, for example, you might want to cover it with a condom. The same is true with most types of food, and should include popsicles and most things frozen. The reason for this is that food may be considered safe for consumption, but we absorb things in our stomach very differently than we do through our skin. In the case of a popsicle, I recommend making your own using a popsicle mold and plain water. This is because those made for the food market, are generally high in sugar and that's not good for your vagina.

Another area where a condom might be advisable is if you and a male partner are partaking in some mutual masturbation. Although the chances of getting pregnant are slim, if there is no actual contact between the two of you, it's easy to get carried away in this situation. Having a condom at the ready can help to avoid the worry of a possible unwanted pregnancy.

Pass Me the Life Jacket Please
Water can provide many areas of pleasure when it comes to solo sex, but it does come with some inherent dangers: drowning being the most obvious. It is possible to drown in under two inches of water, after all. You should always be aware of your surroundings when you are playing with water, in order to prevent mishaps.

One of those mishaps is scalding yourself, and, worse still, scalding your most delicate bits. I'm not sure about you, but in our house, if someone flushes the toilet, decides to do the laundry, or puts on a cup of coffee, the water pressure changes and is something you should be aware of if you are not completely alone in the house. Nothing kills the mood faster than having hot water hit your skin where once there was cool-to-tepid water.

Another pitfall is masturbating when standing in the shower. I like to use silicone lube when I'm playing in the water because of its long-lasting properties, but this can come with an inherent danger. I was once standing in the shower, happily masturbating with my favorite waterproof toy, when suddenly I was hit by an incredibly intense orgasm. I'm not sure whether I slipped on a drop of silicone lube, or whether I simply slipped, but I almost hit my head on the walls of the bathroom. Luckily it was not hard, but it taught me to find a better position and to be careful with drops of lube when I was masturbating in the shower.

Talking of toys, it's worth reminding you that power tools do not belong in the bathroom. I'm talking about the kind of toys that are plugged into the wall outlet here, by the way. They should NEVER be placed in the tub and personally I prefer not to use them in the bathroom at all. Electrocution is not the kind of shock we are looking for here.

Powerful jets can make for powerful orgasms in a spa or swimming pool, but too powerful can cause a lot of pain afterwards. Be aware that when you are playing with strong water jets it's best not to allow the water/air to enter your vagina. Instead, try to concentrate the water onto your clitoris. This will likely give you a far better orgasm. If the jets prove too powerful a sensation for you, consider slipping into the pool or spa with either your costume or a pair of cotton panties on. This can seriously help lessen the risk of soreness afterwards and can often make for a more enjoyable experience during your solo sex session.

Keep Your Feet on the Ground
If you are masturbating in a swimming pool and decide to masturbate by using the outlet jets, try and find a position where you can keep your feet firmly on the bottom of the pool. If this is not possible, you might want to rethink your choice of masturbation tools. If you are still determined to go for the Olympic medal of masturbating in a pool, please be sure to keep one hand on the edge of said pool. Drowning, after all, is rarely sexy, in my experience.

Don't Play With Your Food!
Yes, there are certain foods that are safe to play with externally, but there are many that should never see the inside of your vagina. These include, but are not limited to, popsicles, lollipops,

and basically anything with a high-sugar content. It's also worth repeating that if you do choose to play with a cucumber or zucchini then you should make sure not only is it washed, but if possible use a condom on it.

Stop, Look, and Think Before Proceeding

As I mentioned before, it's so easy to get carried away when you are turned on and just want to scratch an itch that you or someone else may have created. Oftentimes those itches seem to occur when you least expect them or in the most inconvenient of places. Have you ever been driving down the road and been hit by the masturbation bug? I know I have. Sometimes it might be at work, another time it might be at a concert, but generally speaking it happens in a public place. If you can wait to get home to scratch that itch I would, but if not make sure that you are not in danger of finding yourself in a dangerous situation, and, importantly, one that is unlikely to place you into the nearest police cruiser or job center.

Of course, women are in a better position for secret masturbating than their male counterparts, but public masturbation does come with some risks, most of which are obvious. It's maybe okay to discreetly put your hand down your panties and have some fun, but if others can see, you run the risk of causing offence, so be careful.

Don't Masturbate and Drive

Masturbating whilst driving constitutes driving without due care and attention and is similar to texting while driving. It might seem like fun, but it's actually considered very dangerous and can land you in the slammer if you cause an accident. My advice if you want to masturbate on a trip, ask someone else to drive, get a blanket and sit in the back seat. The other option is to find a secluded spot, pull over, and go to town without fear of not reaching your actual destination.

Vibrators Ruin Women for Sex Without Them

Does driving ruin you for walking? No, it just gets you there faster. The same is true for sex with and without vibrators. The vulva, clitoris, nipples, and other parts of the body respond to erotic stimulation no matter where it comes from: fingers, tongues, penises, or vibrators. Vibrators produce the most intense sensations, so most women reach orgasm faster. But using vibrators – even frequently – does not change women's ability to respond to other types of sexual stimulation.

Vibrators can actually *help* women respond to other erotic stimulation. They allow women to experience the full range of their sexual responses, and to become more comfortable with their erotic selves. Greater self-knowledge learned with a vibrator usually helps women respond to other types of sexual play.

When is Too Much Masturbation Too Much?

The simple answer to this question is when it interferes with either a relationship with a partner or your daily life. If you find yourself masturbating rather than seeking out your partner at least some of the time, or you stop going to work or school because you would rather be at home masturbating, then you may have a problem. If this is the case, I would strongly urge you to seek the help of a professional sex therapist.

Masturbation During Pregnancy: Is it safe?

Again the simple answer is, if you are experiencing no problems with your pregnancy, then there is no reason why you should not masturbate. Masturbation is completely natural and safe during pregnancy as long as your doctor hasn't restricted you from such actions.

Conclusion:

If in doubt, please play it safe when it comes to your solo sex sessions. If it appears that a situation or practice may not be safe, the chances are it probably won't be and you risk ending up at the ER. Just because you read it on the Internet does not necessarily mean it's a good idea, either. Sex, especially solo sex, is supposed to be fun, after all. Whilst it can be fraught with dangers, just taking a few simple precautions can turn what might be a disastrous night into a very sexy experience.

CHAPTER 12

Masturbation and Relationships

We tend to think of masturbation as something we do on a purely solo basis. In other words, alone, but it doesn't have to be that way. I know what you're thinking, why would I want to bring someone into my private masturbation world? The answers to that can be many and varied, and often depend upon the length of your relationship, but let's explore the idea together, shall we?

I'm not saying that by any means masturbation is meant to replace partnered sex, but what I am saying is that both can sit side my side and are not mutually exclusive to one another – and neither should they be. Of course, they both have benefits and merits and learning to be comfortable with each of them can be very beneficial to both your physical and emotional wellbeing, and isn't that what we all want?

Mutual Masturbation for Education

Believe it or not, your partner was not born with radar that detects or senses what you enjoy sexually. When you are in a new relationship and ready to move to the next level, it's easy to think that things will just happen naturally and that your new partner will have all the right moves. The truth is often further from the truth than we'd like to admit. Now, this is where mutual masturbation might just come in handy as a practical learning tool.

By now I'm hoping that you are comfortable with your own body and all that it is capable of, and if so, by showing your partner the magic key to your orgasm, you can both benefit, not to mention save a lot of time lost fumbling around in the dark looking for it.

If your partner is more comfortable with showing you how they masturbate first, watch and learn from them. If neither of you is comfortable masturbating first or with another present, then you might want to consider how you communicate with your partner. If you're not comfortable sharing with your partner when you are not intending to touch each other, perhaps you are not comfortable enough to consider partnered sex with that person, even.

Remember, masturbation is a safe form of sexual expression. I've said it before, but I'll say it again, it's hard to get pregnant when you are masturbating! That said, there is a really, really small possibility if you are masturbating with a male partner that you could and it's still wise to take a few precautions. If he comes and then touches your vulva, there is a very distant possibility that you could conceive and, for that reason, I would do one of two things. Either have him wash up after he's come and before he touches you, or ask him to use a condom when he masturbates. Not only is this the safer method, it also makes for an easy clean-up, and who doesn't like that?

That said, mutual masturbation is about the safest form of sexual expression known, and as I said before can be a great learning tool at any point in a relationship. Of course, 'mutual' implies that both parties are masturbating at the same time, but it doesn't have to be that way. There is nothing wrong in simply lying back and letting your partner give you a show, or the other way around. The great thing about being female is that we are capable of more than one orgasm, and whilst this is true for many men as well, remember that they will probably need a break after they have come once. One of the things Hubby and I enjoy doing is watching one another masturbate and then putting into practice what we think we have learned about each other by doing so. There are times when he will masturbate for me, but not come, watch me masturbate and then allow himself to come. There are so many variations of mutual masturbation that to limit yourself to just masturbating together seems, frankly, to be something of a waste.

Another way you can vary the mutual masturbation game is to vary your location. We tend to think that partnered sex should involve a bed, but why not take it outside the bedroom? Consider sitting at either end of the couch, for example, or in opposite kitchen chairs for a change of scene.

Penetrative Sex Might Not Take You Where You Need To Be
We tend to think of penetration as being the ultimate goal of any encounter with a partner, but many women are unable to obtain an orgasm from penetrative sex alone. Many times women require at least some clitoral stimulation in order to achieve an orgasm. Hopefully, you will have a partner who understands that this might be true in your case. If this is not the case and you're finding it difficult to achieve orgasm, you can put all those hours of solo sex to good use and help yourself, so to speak.

For example, if you find yourself unable to reach orgasm via the thrusting movements of your partner, there are no rules that say it's wrong to elect to give yourself a helping hand. If you know that you need clitoral stimulation in order to reach orgasm, and if the opportunity presents itself, you can always use your fingers to mimic the movements that you use during solo sex to stimulate your clitoris the way it needs. If your partner is open to the idea, you can always ask them to help by stimulating your clitoris whilst they enter you as well. If you have masturbated together, they should have some idea of what movements make you happy and, if not, you can both have fun learning.

Why Does He/She Still Masturbate When I'm Ready and Available?

Many of us may feel that once we have found a partner, the need or urge to masturbate will automatically disappear. Nothing could be further from the truth for many of us and there are plenty of instances where masturbation can be a healthy part of a couple's sex life. There will likely be times when your partner is simply unavailable to you; they are maybe traveling for their job or sick, for example. This is a time when masturbation can fill the void created by their absence and rather than looking at masturbation in a negative way, it can be a great time to get back in touch with yourself, quite literally. Over time, people change and so do their sexual needs. It's normal at the beginning of any relationship to act like horny rabbits and take chances, but over the course of a relationship many things are apt to change, just because that's the way life works. We settle down with a partner, perhaps have children, a career, or both, buy a house, and add some more bills into the mix and somewhere along the line sex goes out the window. Now, instead of horny rabbits, you are more like turtles flaying on your back looking for a way to reconnect, and this is often the perfect time to masturbate, perhaps separately at first and then together when you are comfortable doing so.

There are also times in our busy modern-day lives, when simply spending some time alone and masturbating can be relaxing. Orgasms are designed to make you feel good, after all, so a happy masturbator can equate to a happy partner in many cases. Many couples discover, as the years go by, that they also have different sex drives. One might want to have sex more than the other and masturbation is simply a way to bridge the gap for them. It's not a condemnation of you as a sexual partner, but more a need to scratch an itch.

Long-Distance Relationships and Masturbation
Masturbation is the glue that often holds a long-distance relationship together. When you are separated by miles, often physical contact is all but impossible, and so either masturbating together over the phone or a webcam is the only sexual contact that can be made or expected.

Long-distance relationships are, by definition, more challenging than a conventional relationship, but they are by no means any less valid. One advantage of a long- distance relationship is that it allows each member of the partnership time to get to know one another. As there is no, or little, actual physical contact, exploring your partner's mind and fantasies can become a great way to get to know them better. Masturbation should become the natural outlet for your fantasies and desires. Of course, you will have to overcome the social stigmas that society puts on masturbation, but this can be a good thing, in my book. Learning to love yourself whilst you learn to love someone else can be a powerful experience if you open your mind to it.

Laptops, Cell Phones, and Vibes. Oh My!
If you are in a long-distance relationship then you will likely be aware that masturbation is your lifeline. It's hard to have sex with someone who lives even 100 miles down the road, but technology and masturbation are your friends here. Even if you are not in a long-distance relationship it can be fun to combine technology and masturbation with a partner for some fun. Let me explain a little more.

175

I'm old enough to recall a time when sex was something that was always done in person, so to speak. Of course, back in the good old days we had phones, but horror upon horror, many were connected by a wire to the base. I know! Imagine that! I can also remember the very first cell phones, which, for the most part, resembled a large brick – good for hitting a potential assailant if calling 911 was not an option, but not so conducive with phone sex. I tried it once, and as I recall the brick was really heavy and I enjoyed a two-handed technique back then which was almost impossible to do without spending weeks at the gym beforehand. So why am I telling you this, you might ask? The reason is simple, we live in a world filled with technology and there is no reason on this earth why you should not incorporate that technology into your sex life as well relationship, and also your masturbation routines.

Laptops and cell phones have opened up a new world when it comes to masturbation and, trust me when I tell you that if you want to masturbate with your cell phone, there is an app for that! Yes, there really is! In fact, there are several apps that will be happy to help you utilize the vibration mode on your cell phone. There are even some apps that will help your partner utilize the vibration mode, believe it or not. Over the years I've tried a few of these apps and, to be honest, it's much more fun to simply set your cell phone to vibrate or get your partner to call you and call you. You can have fun with your partner this way, and after you've recovered from an orgasm, enjoy a long conversation about what turned you on and what didn't.

'I masturbate a lot, since I am in a long-distance relationship. Often, I make myself really wet by thinking erotic thoughts or talking dirty with my boyfriend on the phone. Then, I lie face-down on my bed. I lie on top of my right hand and put my middle finger right on top of my clit. Without moving my finger and using my own wetness as lubricant, simply just hump my finger. While doing it, I often

imagine that someone (sometimes a woman) is going down on me.
I come really quickly using this technique.'

Another fun way to use your cell phone is to use the video capability it has. Just a word of caution here, though: NEVER send a video of yourself masturbating to someone you do not know well. Once a video is out there, it's very difficult, actually almost impossible, to dial it back in. If you do not trust the person you are sending it to 100 per cent or have even an inkling of doubt, my advice is don't press send. That said, videoing yourself can be an added turn-on and is a great way to get comfortable with masturbating and watching yourself masturbate. There is nothing wrong with sharing the video with your partner. I would just wait to do that in person, if possible, that way you keep the evidence in your possession, so to speak. Once watched, I would advise deleting the video, as there is nothing more embarrassing than having to explain to your brother the video you sent out by mistake and if you think I'm being dramatic, it has happened before and the results were not pretty for anyone involved.

Many couples enjoy watching each other masturbate in real time via their laptops and a third-party video service such as Skype or even snap chat. Whilst both of these and the many other similar apps on the market have their place, always make sure you completely trust the other person before you consider doing this.

When I first discovered masturbation, sex toys were little more than a piece of plastic, shaped like a penis, and with a motor that made it buzz. Boy, have we come a long way since then, thankfully! Nowadays the selection of toys available can be overwhelming, and this is coming from someone who tests and reviews sex toys almost every day. The toys that are making technological break-throughs, such as the OhMiBod company, are on the cutting edge of masturbation technology. Toys like those made by OhMiBod can be synced up with your i-pod and will pulsate to the music you are listening to, but great strides are being made in this area and there are new products being brought onto the market on a daily basis that promise to amp up your sex life via technology. Some of these include things such as two devices, one for each partner, and an app that controls each device. Each partner then has complete control over the other device and can cause it to vibrator-pulsate at their whim via the app. There is even an entire body suit that has been developed with the idea that both partners can control and experience sex whilst in entirely different countries, but at the time of writing this is still in development and the manufacturers are trying to figure out how to make it affordable for the average couple.

If you've ever watched the film *The Ugly Truth* you will likely remember the scene where Mike gives Abby her first vibrator and then proceeds to take her to dinner with the boss and treats her to an evening of orgasmic bliss. If you want to replicate this evening, you might want to invest in a pair of vibrating panties that are remotely controlled. Give your partner the remote control and tell them they are in control for the night. The results can be very satisfying.

Conclusion:
Masturbation can be a healthy part of a relationship and if your partner chooses to masturbate occasionally, then I say either leave them to it or join in the fun. The only time that masturbation could be viewed as a problem within an otherwise healthy relationship is if it is taking the place of sex with your partner. For example, if you find yourself masturbating to web porn rather than making love to your partner each night you might want to reconnect with them on a more physical basis. The bottom line here, though, is that masturbation can be a healthy form of sexual expression no matter where you are in a relationship and it should be viewed as such.

CHAPTER 13

The Bottom Line

If you've reached this part of the book, then I would like to first congratulate you and just say I hope that you have found value in what you have read.

When I began this book, I had no idea how large or small it would be, but I did know a couple of things – masturbation is not just about the way in which you choose to stimulate your genitals. It's so much more than that, as I hope you have realized. Masturbation, just like any sexual act, begins in the mind, and often long before any part of a person's body may have been touched. It encompasses so many things that we often don't even consider. It's a complicated beast, just like its partnered alternative. Just as there is no right way to have sex, there is no way right way to masturbate – just *your* way. The main difference lies in the fact that masturbation really is all about what works for you. No partner means that the only person you have to please, or learn to please sexually, is yourself.

Masturbation can also be considered a very low-pressure sexual

179

act if you stop to think about it. By virtue of the fact that there is no partner watching you, and in some cases judging you, it can be a freeing sexual experience; one that allows you to learn what works for you sexually, without that pressure, and it's a great way to explore your own sexual self.

This can be a fun journey if you allow yourself to start going down the path. There will likely be times of change in your life. Times you may find yourself without a partner for a number of reasons, times when you are simply too busy to consider partnered sex, but still get horny. Having a tried-and-tested way to scratch that horny itch can save you from making some bad, and occasionally life-altering, decisions.

Over the years, my own masturbation habits have changed and adapted to fit in with the changes that have occurred in my own life. I've also grown sexually and experimented, thanks in no small part, to Clitical.com. I love to read other women's sexual fantasies, masturbation techniques, and even now I am often surprised when a new technique hits the site, or a different and unique variation of a tried-and-tested technique is shared. I love the fact that women feel safe enough in the space that I have created to, in fact, share what is often a most intimate experience for them. By sharing with others, we have the potential to expand everyone's knowledge of female sexuality, and especially masturbation techniques and all they entail.

I hope as you have read this book, you too have become more comfortable with the idea of masturbation. I would love one day for masturbation to be seen for what it actually is, a creatively sexual learning tool as opposed to the ugly step sister of partnered sex. I think we are moving closer to that time, but we still have a way to go as a society until masturbation is completely out from under the covers.

Until that time comes, I will leave you with some of the creative ways that Clitical's visitors have learned to celebrate their own bodies and all the pleasure they can give you. I hope that they inspire you to do the same!

Happy masturbating!

CHAPTER 14

Real Masturbation Technique as Told by Clitical.com Visitors

Over the past 15 years we have had a lot of techniques that have been submitted by Clitical visitors. What I decided to do for this book is to categorize them by the techniques that have proved most popular over those years. Apart from that, they are in no particular order and many are submitted anonymously or with pen names. I hope you enjoy this selection of techniques from real women from around the world.

Bathroom Divas:
'I do this sometimes when I need a quick orgasm. In the bathroom I take a bath towel and place it over the edge of the counter of the sink. This provides padding. I sometimes take my underwear off, but I usually leave it on. I stand so that I am facing the counter. The counter edge is a few inches higher than my clit. I put the palms of my hands on the edge of the counter and prop myself up so my feet are off the floor. I press the area above my clit against the counter with the towel between my body and the counter as a cushion. I lean forward a little and rock back

and forth just slightly. My entire body weight is centered right on the area above my clit (not the tip because that would be too sensitive), so I am able to put a lot of pressure there. You have to find the right spot or else it is uncomfortable. I do this and, usually within two minutes or less, I have the most intense orgasm. It looks dorky but it feels amazing!

I discovered this by accident one time when I was really young. I was leaning over a railing and felt a wonderful sensation in my genitals. I did not know what it was and I did not even know what masturbation was then (I was, like, seven or eight). I started doing this in other places – wherever I could find something higher than my waist to lift myself up and push against (the side of the sofa, back of chairs, washing machine, dresser, end of my bed, and, of course, the sink). I would always do this through whatever clothing I had on. Eventually, I started having orgasms while doing this and got to the point where I would take everything off except my underwear (when nobody was home, of course). I always thought that I must be weird and that nobody else did this. It was always my own little special secret.'

'I only started masturbating a few months ago, which, I know, is unusual for an 18-year-old. I read on the Cosmopolitan website that someone had an orgasm by positioning herself under the running water of her bathtub and I decided to give it a shot. Low and behold, it felt really great and I have been doing it ever since. I'm not sure, but it may not be a good idea to have water entering the body, so I use this for clitoral stimulation only, making sure to get as little as possible inside of me. Give this a try next time you're in the tub, you won't be sorry... unless the water is too hot.'

'Standing up can provide two types of orgasms. I like to lean against the wall across from the bathroom sink and put a foot on the sink top. This is a good position to reach the g-spot. When I find the spot, fluid flows rapidly, this is what I call the "little O". After I have the little O, stimulating my clitoris brings me close to what I call the "big O", but, like the others, I enjoy backing off a little until I just can't stand it any more. When I starting rubbing my clit again, I pretend that someone else is in control and do not stop for anything. This causes a huge orgasm.'

Water Babies:
'This is my first post to the site after a long time of reading and getting horny. My first method I discovered at a very young age. My cousin and I used to sit in my grandparents' hot tub with the jets turned on to full pressure. We would lie up against the side so we wouldn't get our hair wet, but we soon realized that the water shooting out of the jets kind of "tickled". The intense pressure of the water on our clits was enough to make us squirm when we were about eight years old. I loved the feeling so much that I now use a shower head on massage mode.'

'I have only recently begun to masturbate and I love to read the stories and techniques on this site. One of my favorite ways to masturbate requires a bit of time. I can orgasm by just rubbing my clit, but that's boring after a while. After reading some of these stories, I get in the tub and get the water running to a good temperature. I position my clit right under the stream of water, the harder the better. I take my hands and spread my lips open, so the water hits my clit directly. This gets me off pretty quickly, but the most intense orgasm I've ever had came after that. After the first orgasm, I let the water keep running, then my climax builds slowly. The feeling is amazing. Instead of spastic jerking and shaking, your entire body trembles, and I have no control. Amazing, but requires some time and an empty house (it can get loud!).'

'I like to use a hand-held shower massage and lean back against

the wall, letting the water stream on my pussy. It's incredible –
like a bunch of tiny tongues licking at me all at once. I live alone
and masturbation helps both relieve tension, put me in touch with
someone I wish were touching me, and, above all, gives such a good
feeling. I've tried many "things", but what's most available are my
own two hands. Using one on my breasts/one on my clitoris – that
makes for a climax every time!'

'I love to masturbate and can masturbate forever. First I become
naked and lie on my stomach on my bed. (Before doing this, I
keep some ice cubes ready.) I rub them on my naked body. The
ice cubes make my body wet. Now since I am wet, I then imagine
that I am a fish who has been caught. I then do all the actions
that a fish does when taken out of water i.e. I hump and rock
my body back and forth on my bed. I explode soon and cum.
Oh, I gotta go and do this now!'

'First, I usually watch some hardcore porn or some lesbian porn to
make myself horny. Then, I get in the shower and adjust my shower
head until it's one pulsating flow, then I try different positions – on
my back with legs spread, on my knees sitting up, on my knees with
one hand holding the shower head and one on the ground, sitting
on the edge of the tub, lying on my side with my leg in the air, I've
even tried standing up, then I put the flowing water onto my hard
clit, and sometimes move it up and down and WOW! I get horny
thinking about it. I get the best orgasms EVER from this, moaning,
screaming, breathless orgasm. It's FABULOUS!'

'First I read a very erotic book or magazine while in the bathtub,
then I let the water flow at a very slow rate and lie on my back
(the water level is fairly low) and place my genital area under the
water flow. I use one hand, usually the left, to "open" the area,
then lie back and fantasize! The results are great! Sometimes I
use the ribbed end of my hairbrush if I feel like I need a little

185

more, or if I am really frustrated. Also a hand-held shower head with a real fast pulsating stream works great!'

'Here's another technique women might like to try. I recently found that if you fill a long balloon with water and freeze it you will have a toy that will play for a long time and when you're finished you can refreeze it till you need it again. The sensation of the cold melting inside you is incredible, and the shape is about the same as an erect cock, which makes that much more enjoyable. My husband loves to watch me masturbate with it and lick the ice-cold juices from me afterwards.'

'Recently I've been getting bored with doing the same stuff so I read online it's AMAZING to use your shower head it has to be detachable though and since I didn't have that I used my bathtub faucet instead and omg it was AMAZING here's what I did.

I properly positioned myself under it but most importantly I check and make sure the water is a good warmth but not too hot then position myself under and the water is so soft and gentle yet so powerfully when it hits your clit it's AMAZING the pre orgasms I get are just great and I can't help from screaming the great thing about this is I don't have to spend money and its DISCRETE unless you make a mess ... you can change the pulse of the water and I find when I bend my head back it feels good to be careful if you're going to let the water fill the tub I don't ... but if you want to make sure you don't drown lol I usually do this after my shower and when you're done sometimes you can't walk my legs shake when it feels good try it you won't be upset.'

Improvised Toys:
'My favorite sex toy in the world is a vibrator! I use my friends whenever I am at her house. When I am at home alone all I want is to have a vibrator inside me! So one day as I was home alone

cleaning my room I was naked and extremely horny! Just teasing myself and playing with my pussy. Until i came across my new Venus razor that vibrates! I opened it up turned it on and placed it on my throbbing wet pussy and it feels so good! Just as good as a vibrator! Now I fuck myself with it all the time!!!(; and it gives the best orgasms EVER!'

'First I wait until everyone has gone out, then I take my electric toothbrush and Venus Gillette razor and sit on the computer chair. I read through the masturbation techniques submitted at Clitical.com, then browse my favorite porn site. I watch a couple of girl-on-girl porn movies and insert the handle of the razor into my pussy. I sit back and hold the electric toothbrush over my clit but not under my panties. I sit back and watch the movie with one hand pumping the razor handle in and out of my pussy, hitting my g-spot. I use my other hand to keep the electric toothbrush in the right place. When I have nearly reached orgasm I switch off the electric toothbrush and pull out the razor handle and allow my body to recover. Then I start all over again. I repeat this about three times until I reach an amazing orgasm that lasts for ages. If you don't have an electric toothbrush, you can use any vibrator or your hand.'

'Masturbating with shower heads and vibrators always left me feeling somewhat empty. I wanted something closer to the real thing! I use Polish sausages. I found some very thin-skinned Polish sausages at my local supermarket. They are about eight inches long and four inches in diameter. I take one and heat it slowly in warm water until it is warm all the way through. Then I gently slide it into my vagina. I'm already wet with anticipation and use it just like a real penis. It's warm and the rigidity is perfect. The sensation is beyond description. Sometimes I can postpone my climax for up to an hour and it is HEAVEN! Sometimes I keep another one in a pan of warm water ready if the one I am using breaks or cools off.'

187

'I've just turned 18, but have been masturbating since I was 14. When I get home the first thing I do is get semi naked and pleasure myself with my fingers, but after my first orgasm I find it hard to get to my second. Ladies I'm telling you toothbrushes are the way forward. I put that baby on full power and within 30 seconds my pussy juice is running down my thighs and I'm desperate for more!'

'I used to use an electric flosser that I had. It is small and quiet and does the job really well, but I noticed that the battery was getting low and the vibration wasn't as strong. Then I remembered the electric toothbrush I had just gotten. As soon as I stuck it to my clit I was moaning. I orgasmed fast and just keep doing it over and over.'

'After reading about using an electric toothbrush masturbation technique, I decided to try it out myself with a few modifications. Since I have a sensitive clit myself, I place a small towel (like a face cloth) over my vagina first. Then, using the bristled side of the electric toothbrush (the other side doesn't have as powerful vibrations and tends to get hot), I let it go all over my clit, occasionally running it over my lips and hole. The feeling is amazing and the orgasms even better! And, best of all, it's fast and anyone in the house will think you've just been brushing your teeth for a while if they hear anything.'

'Last night I was reading some of the Clitical stories and some of your techniques and I found myself slowly beginning to strip (I find taking my clothes off piece by piece makes my clit beg to be touched even more, which really gets me going). My usual technique is to grab my Oral-B electric toothbrush and start it at my nipples and then slowly move it down my body and around my clit, until I can't resist any more. I put it on my clit and have a mind-blowing orgasm. I always picture a girl licking my soaking-wet pussy. I have a major turn-on when it comes to girl-on-girl. I never have been with one, but have truly always dreamed of it.

But instead I was craving something different…I have recently enjoyed watching squirting videos, they drive me wild. I began watching some last night and thinking of having such an amazing orgasm. I simply had to try… I slowly slipped my fingers in and began fingering myself like never before and loving every second of it. At one point I got a bit frustrated because every time I thought I was getting close nothing happened. I kept trying and thought of the technique I had seen in the videos where women rub their pussy side to side really fast. THAT WORKED! Just as I felt myself about to cum I started rubbing my pussy as hard and fast as I could. I was squirting everywhere. I simply couldn't stop. I wanted more and more each time. It was the most fabulous feeling. I found myself letting go to the point where I was rubbing my juices all over my ass and legs and licking my fingers one by one to taste myself. Thinking about it again now makes me want to do it again right this second. I stood up off of my bed and felt drips of juices running down my legs, it was the most satisfying feeling. I couldn't help but smile… I went to bed feeling so happy and complete. I am going to go do it again right now!

So my techniques basically are: Oral-B electric brush (tease yourselves, ladies, it makes it much more satisfying), fingering: while doing this to try and make yourself squirt, make sure you are focusing only on the g-spot. Make your fingers hook into your vagina and simply do the "come here" motion with those two fingers… keep working at it. It may take a while, so try not to get frustrated! When you feel yourself start to tense up and your g-spot becomes hard, press on it a few more times and then do the rubbing side to side really fast and really hard (keep pushing with your insides, it's all about the push and the tension). I hope this works for some of you.

P.S. When trying to squirt, try to be in a comfortable spot, BUT make sure you put a towel under you so it doesn't make a mess on your sheets!'

189

'My last masturbation session happened after midnight in my room. I was wearing thin pajamas and no bra. I started off by reading female techniques to get myself hot. While reading, I started by caressing my nipples. Before I knew it, I was pinching them and started to feel my vagina tingly and very wet. I took off my shorts, put my hands in my panties, and started running my fingers up and down my labia. After that, I took off my panties and top and circled my clit and then, with my wetness, pinched my nipples again. When I couldn't take it any more I laid on the floor and with a fat marker I pressed my clitoris. I started to rock my hips back and forth, squeezed, and came.'

Humping Good Fun:
'So I just recently discovered the fun that I can have with my body pillow! I place it on the floor, lie on top of it, and place my legs on either side and hump it just a little to get the juices flowing. After, I read a few stories on here or go into a chat room, then I begin to hump it faster. Today, I took a water bottle and filled it with cold water and placed it right underneath me and began to hump that. Let me tell you, between the cool temp of the water and the ridges on the bottle, it felt great! Let me know what other things you would place on the pillow to hump…'

'I like to sit with my legs bent to where the lower half of my leg is touching the floor, take a pillow and ride it for a bit. Then I make a fist, pressing my knuckle where my clit is (with the pillow still there) and fuck like mad! The first time I ever came was doing that.'

'I've been masturbating for a long time and over the years my favorite has been to grind my pillow. I have tried other things and I do enjoy them, but I just love humping my pillow. It just gives me the best orgasms ever. What I like to do is to put my pillowcases in the freezer (in a bag, so it won't touch anything else) and keep it in there so it can get nice and cold. After a while, you place it back onto your pillow and you grind away. It

190

is kinda weird at first, but I grew to love it as the coldness runs up my hot thighs as I start to heat it up. Hope someone will try this and let me know how it goes.'

'Stack three pillows up on top of each other on your floor or your bed. Then put down something to cover the pillow on top, because you will get wet, I guarantee it. Get a t-shirt/washcloth/towel and roll it up hot-dog style. Get naked, at least your bottom half and hump away. Feels soo good...'

'I'm a very happily married mother of ten (believe it or not!). My husband and I have been married for 25 years this year and we are expecting our first grandchild. Our sex life has been good and healthy (obvious from the number of children!). As we've gotten older, we still have great sex, but with the understandable stresses of a large family and work, and life in general, we only have sex about one or two times a week now. Often we are just tired at the end of the day. We are often tired enough that just holding hands in bed or spooning is comfortable on those nights we don't have sex. But I still want sexual satisfaction other times, and so...

About twice a week after the kids are off to school and I get back from the gym from working out, before I shower, I get naked and pull back the sheets on the bed. We have king-sized pillows that are really springy. I love the luscious feeling of the cool sheets on my body, especially because I'm usually warm from working out. I lie flat on my stomach and play with my nipples with one or both hands as I press against the mattress and as I spread my legs wide apart and then back tightly together across the sheets. It usually doesn't take long until I'm really horny and then I grab one of our pillows and put it between my legs. Then I keep lying flat on my stomach and occasionally roll up on my side as I grind against the springy pillow. The feeling against my clit is just the best and I always have an incredible climax

191

in only a minute or two. Then I have a hot shower and steam myself for 30 minutes. What a start to a great day!'

'I almost always start masturbating my playing with my nipples because this never fails to get me nice and worked up. I have a lot of methods for masturbating, but this one I call the "pillow method". I put one pillow between my legs and hump it while I stack others up under my chest and rub my tits on them. My cunt always gets incredibly wet and I like the feeling of rubbing that wetness all over the pillow. (I usually use my husband's pillow, because the thought of him getting a nice whiff of my juices when he gets into bed later turns me on.) I like looking at my nipples as I rub them against the pillow, too... Before you know it, here I CUM!'

Boudoir Babes:
'As I lie here in my tub, water steaming, bubbles surrounding me, my pussy starts to ache. I caress my body, fondle my boobs, and pinch my nipples. My hand slides down, and I slip one finger into my moist pussy and rub my clit as I slowly slide my finger in and out.

I get out of the tub, make my way to my bedroom, and slip into my silk sheets completely naked. I'm now beginning to lose self control as lust takes over. My pussy, now dripping wet, longing for attention, aches with the need to be touched and satisfied. I toss and turn and rub my body against my sheets, my wetness dripping onto it.'

Public Masturbators:
'Last year I went through a horrible divorce, which I'm not going to elaborate on. Suffice to say I'm now single again and, to be honest, not actively looking for somebody else. If anybody has read my previous posts on this website they will know I like both men and women, but at this moment in time I need my own space.

However, being on my own means I've been masturbating... A LOT. Plus I've been watching a fair bit of porn, too, and found a video of an Australian girl having a wank in the changing rooms of a clothes shop. The video is so hot and I wondered what it would be like to copy her.

The thought of frigging myself off and cumming next to somebody innocently trying on clothes and the danger of being caught intrigued me. The first couple of times I chickened out, but now I'm practically doing it all the time.

At first I copied the girl on the video I saw. I tried on completely new clothes with the security and price tags still on them. For obvious reasons the shops don't like you trying on knickers, but I'd sneak them in. Call me perverse, but the thought of soaking a pair of knickers and putting them back on the shelf for another customer to buy made me feel so horny and nasty.

I only did that a few times. I now like to do it in front of the full-length mirrors, completely naked apart from new pair of shoes.

I've tried it in loads of places. My favorites are the changing rooms with curtains down corridors. I used to like them because you can see out (and in) where the curtains don't quite close properly BUT now I like them for a whole new reason.

Last week I went to my favorite place. Picked up a few clothes with absolutely no intention of trying them on and a pair of stilettos. There was nobody in the cubicles, so I went in the one at the very end, stripped off, and put my new shoes on. I stood with my legs slightly apart and started to gently stroke myself.

Soon I was wet and ready. I fingered my soaking pussy with my left hand whilst rubbing my clit with my right.

Pretty soon I was getting close. Then a moment of madness came over me. I stopped and listened but couldn't hear anybody. I turned and opened the curtain fully and turned back to finish wanking myself off in front of the mirror.

I came immediately and nearly collapsed. My heart was beating and my pussy was soaking and throbbing. Stifling my orgasm was tough and I quickly drew the curtain back. I do find it strange that when I'm masturbating, I'm somewhat brazen and reckless, but as soon as I've cum I immediately become shy again.

This was one of the most memorable orgasms I've had ever. The only thing I wish I could've done differently is if I'd had my butt plug in too. But at least having that option still available to me gives me something to look forward to.

Anyway, this is my new technique and I wanted to share it with you all. I hope if any of you try it you'll enjoy it as much as I do. For me it brings a whole new meaning to the phrase "retail therapy".

'The first time I ever masturbated in public was at the gym. To make a long story short, I was staying with my sister for a few days and at the time she lived with a bunch of roommates. Well, whoever was responsible for paying the water bill didn't do so. Luckily, my sister had a gym membership so we were able to take showers there. Being the horny person that I am, I decided that this was the perfect time to have an orgasm or two. It was nerve-wracking, yet exciting at the same time. I was in the shower stall with the hot water running down my back, trying to hold my breath so my moans didn't echo throughout the locker room. After catching my breath I walked out and no one had any idea.'

'Last night I masturbated topless with a bullet vibe down my jeans while in the car driving on the freeway (I was on the passenger side).'

Toy With Me:
'Right after a shower, I lie down on the bed. I use pillows to support my legs. I lube my vibrator and start to swirl it around on my clit. I use one hand on the vibrator and the other to hold open my pussy. I like to change the pressure that I apply to vary the intensity. I do really enjoy my husband taking my breast in his mouth and sucking like a baby. When I get close to my orgasm, I start to feel small ripples of pleasure going through me. As I cum, I call out my husband's name. I lay back and enjoy.'

'Two of my girlfriends and I decided to get a vibrator because we're

194

all single and tired of fruitlessly mingling. We went to a sex shop in Boston and all three got the same vibrator. WOW! I looove it! It only takes one AA battery AND it's waterproof.

So I got home and no one was home – YES! I went to my room and laid on my bed and already started humping the mattress. I look up some lesbian porn – tribbing is my favorite. I lay in my bed and watched and watched and I could feel my pussy lips swelling up and my clit pulsing and my panties getting drenched in my sticky juices.

I grabbed the vibrator from my bag, tore it out the packaging, and ran to the bathroom to wash it. I came back to my room and threw myself in the bed. I ran my hands over my body and felt my nipples poking at my bra. I rubbed my pussy thru my panties and it felt sooo good. I removed all my clothes but my panties. I cranked my vibe to the highest setting and put that thing right in my clit– mmmm – the vibrations drive my pussy crazy and my legs open wide against my will. One hand held the toy and the other was grabbing and squeezing the pillow because it feels oh so good. My eyes are closed and my breath is quickening, my hips are gyrating and slightly raised off the bed, wanting more and more of the goodness.

With my free hand, I rewound the tribbing video, put my headphones on. WOW! Imagine lying on your bed, vibe on your clit and hearing lesbians moaning while they grind their gooey wet pussies together, yum! Their moans excite me more and more. I took the vibe and glide thru my wetness, and, boy, I am dripping wet! I took some of it and rubbed it on my clittie with the vibe and it feels soooo mm mm good that breath caught in my throat. Then I dipped the whole five inches inside myself while the lesbians moaned louder.

I turned my head to see one of them on top, back arched, eyes closed and pussies grinding against her partners. I pumped that vibe in and out like a maniac! I'm really tight so the fiction of the silicone mixed with the vibrations feel like nothing on this earth.

I took the vibe out my wet pussy, opened my pussy lips wide with my free hand and rub the slick vibe on my love button. MMMM I was moaning and groaning like crazy, wishing it was a hot girl's clittie rubbing against mine and I came so hard that I squirted on my bed. I love masturbation

And dang. Writing this for you just made me so hot that my clit is throbbing and begging already and I am squeezing my thighs together mmmm....'

Resources

Blogger and Sex Toy Reviewers:

Clitical.Com
www.clitical.com
Information regarding female masturbation, sex toy reviews and erotica.

Property of Potter
www.propertyofpotter.com
Here you will find sex toy reviews, thoughts on sexuality and a whole lot more.

CaraSutra
www.carasutra.co.uk
This UK based blogger reviews the latest adult products, and has a kinky side you will enjoy.

Dangerous Lilly
www.dangerouslilly.com
Another sex toy reviewing blogger who tells it like it is and is an advocate for safer sex.

Kinkly.Com
www.kinkly.com
A great place with a sex positive attitude that invites sex bloggers to post their thoughts.

There are many, many other sex bloggers out there that offer something for everyone.

Places To Buy Sex Toys, Books And More:
Adam & Eve
www.adamandeve.com
Mail order and online store.

Babeland
www.babeland.com
Sex positive retail and on-line store, located in Seattle and New York.

Come As You Are
www.comeasyouare.com
Sex positive retail and online sex toy company with store in Toronto.

Good Vibrations
www.goodvibes.com
Female friendly and sex positive retail and online store. Locations in San Francisco, Oakland, Berkeley, and Boston.

JTStockroom
www.stockroom.com
JT offers a good selection of BDSM gear for the more adventurous sex positive consumer. Retail and Online stores. Located in Los Angeles.

Lovehoney.Com
www.lovehoney.com
An online adult store, sex positive and female friendly.

Nomia Adult Botique
http://www.nomiaboutique.com
Female friendly and sex positive store in Portland, Maine.

She Bop
www.sheboptheshop.com
Sex positive store with retail location in Portland, Oregon.

General Information
Sexuality About.Com
www.sexuality.about.com
Excellent information on a wide range of sexuality topics.

The American Association of Sexuality Educators, Counselors, and Therapists.
www.aasect.org
If you are looking for a sex therapist, this is the place to start your search.

Planned Parenthood
www.plannedparethood.com
A great place to find all you need to know about STDs, risks and how to avoid them.

www.ingramcontent.com/pod-product-compliance
Lightning Source LLC
Chambersburg PA
CBHW011829020426
42334CB00027B/2991